INTERMEDIATE
Nutrition
& Health

An introduction to the subject of food, nutrition and health

Dr Mabel Blades
PhD, SRD, MBA, BSc, MPhil, DMS, FRSH, FIFST
Registered Public Health Nutritionist & Dietitian

PUBLISHED BY
© HIGHFIELD.CO.UK LTD

'Vue Pointe', Spinney Hill, Sprotbrough,
Doncaster, DN5 7LY, UK
Tel: +44 0845 2260350
Facsimile: +44 0845 2260360
E-mail: richard@highfield.co.uk

Websites:
www.highfield.co.uk
www.foodsafetytrainers.co.uk

ISBN 1 904544 43 6

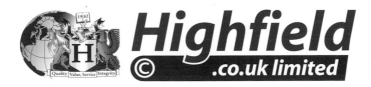

INTERMEDIATE NUTRITION & HEALTH

Dedication

My parents Mabel and Jack Thomason who gave me an enthusiasm for studying and my husband Peter Blades for encouragement to put pen to paper.

First published 2004
2nd Edition 2005

© **HIGHFIELD.CO.UK.LTD**

ISBN 1 904544 43 6

Printed by Trafford Press • Telephone: 01302 367509

Contents

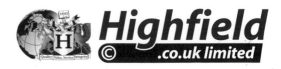

Foreword

The evidence suggests that changes in food habits can lead to significant improvements in health is a key statement by the Food Standards Agency, which is an independent agency set up by an Act of Parliament in 2000 to protect the public's health and consumer interests in relation to food.

A knowledge of nutrition and health is of supreme importance, especially for anyone involved in providing food or any form of care to individuals or groups.

Intermediate Nutrition and Health is an ideal text for use on Intermediate Nutrition and Health courses and to support specialist in-house nutrition courses. It has been developed to take the reader effortlessly through a complex subject. It provides a good, comprehensive basis for anyone wanting to study the subject with easy-to-assimilate sections which are enlivened by memorable illustrations.

Richard A Sprenger
BSc(Hons), DMS, FCIEH, MREHIS, FSOFHT
Managing Director, Highfield.co.uk limited

Preface

Diet and good health

Good health is of supreme importance to us all. It does not matter whether we are the busy mother caring for a family, a business executive or a retired couple: without good health we cannot function as we should like to be able to.

For centuries it has been recognised that what we eat can affect our health. Nowadays research on diet and health confirms that what we eat has a marked effect on how we feel as well as preventing heath problems. Good nutrition is absolutely vital to health, and a good understanding of food, nutrition and health is especially important to anyone involved in the provision of food or health care.

Aims

This book aims to provide information on nutrition, food and diet in relation to health and well-being.

The information in the book covers that required for both basic and intermediate courses in nutrition and health.

Nutrition qualifications such as those of the Royal Society for the Promotion of Health (RSPH) and the Royal Institute of Public Health (RIPH) can provide an invaluable introduction to the subject. As accredited courses they can form part of any portfolio of learning hours.

This 2nd edition has been undertaken due to the recent developments in nutrition and health.

Dr Mabel Blades
PhD, SRD, MBA, BSc, MPhil, DMS, FRSH, FIFST

Dr Mabel Blades is a State Registered Dietitian and Nutritionist.
She regularly writes and broadcasts on nutritional issues,
and has a wealth of expertise in lecturing in this field.

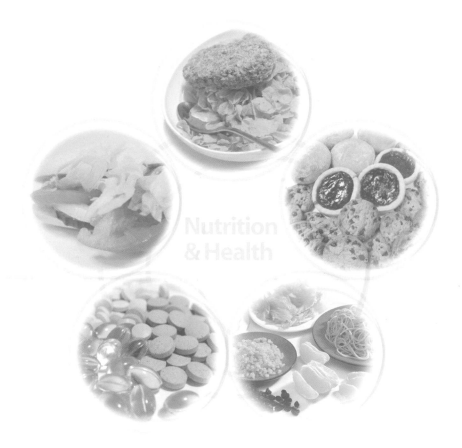

1 Food, nutrition and health

Nutrition is absolutely vital to health, and a good understanding of food, nutrition and health is especially important to anyone involved in the provision of food or health care.

Although the word diet has become synonymous with a slimming diet, in the context of the study of nutrition it means the normal foods and beverages consumed each day.

Food and nutrition

Food
Solid or liquid which supplies energy.
Material for growth, repair and reproduction.
Substances necessary to regulate production of energy release or growth, repair and reproduction.

Nutrition
Study of processes of growth maintenance and repair of the living body which depends upon the digestion and absorption of food.

Diet
Foods and beverages in the amounts eaten.

Background to a healthy diet

It is generally recognised that there are no unhealthy foods, only unbalanced and therefore unhealthy diets. There is general consensus among experts about a diet for health. The Food Standards Agency (FSA) has adopted 'Eight Guidelines for a Healthy Diet':

1. enjoy your food;
2. eat a variety of different foods;
3. eat the right amount to be a healthy weight;
4. eat plenty of foods rich in starch and fibre;
5. eat plenty of fruit and vegetables;
6. don't eat too many foods that contain a lot of fat;
7. don't have sugary foods and drinks too often; and
8. if you drink alcohol drink sensibly.

These 'Eight Guidelines for a Healthy Diet' were previously devised by the Health Education Authority (HEA), Department of Health (DoH) and Ministry of Agriculture, Fisheries and Food (MAFF). (MAFF has been replaced by the Department for the Environment and Rural Affairs (DEFRA) and the HEA by the Health Development Agency).

The Balance of Good Health was originally developed by the HEA but has now been adopted by the Food Standards Agency (FSA) and the Health Development Agency as a model for a healthy diet. The Balance of Good Health is a pictorial illustration of a well-balanced and healthy diet. It shows the five main food groups and the proportions of each of the foods that are recommended to be eaten as part of a healthy diet.

These food groups include:
♦ fruit and vegetables;
♦ bread, other cereals and potatoes;
♦ milk and dairy foods;
♦ meat, fish and alternatives; and
♦ foods containing fat and foods containing sugar.

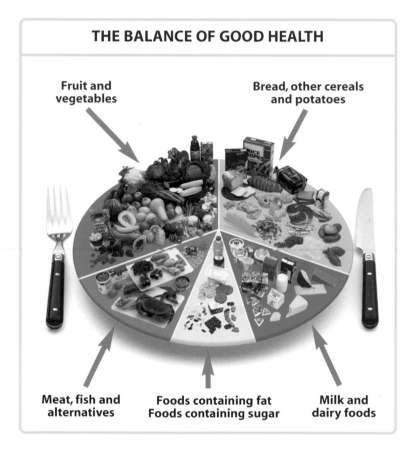

THE BALANCE OF GOOD HEALTH

Fruit and vegetables

Bread, other cereals and potatoes

Meat, fish and alternatives

Foods containing fat Foods containing sugar

Milk and dairy foods

As can be seen from the illustration of the Balance of Good Health, the largest proportions of food that should be eaten as part of a healthy diet are fruit and vegetables and bread, other cereals and potatoes.

The Balance of Good Health focuses on food not nutrients but in general the five food groups contain the following nutrients:
♦ fruit and vegetables - provide vitamins, minerals, some dietary fibre or non-starch polysaccharide (NSP) and carbohydrate;
♦ bread, other cereals and potatoes - provide carbohydrate of a starchy type, some dietary fibre or NSP, especially if these are unrefined foods, vitamins, minerals and protein;
♦ milk and dairy foods - provide protein and vitamins and minerals particularly

MAJOR HEALTH PROBLEMS

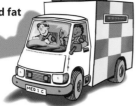

- Coronary heart disease
  - **multifactorial**
  - **diet – saturated fat**
  - **antioxidants**
  - **obesity**
  - **smoking**
  - **exercise**
  - **hypertension**

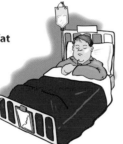

- Cancers
  - **multifactorial**
  - **diet - saturated fat**
  - **antioxidants**
  - **obesity**
  - **smoking**
  - **NSP/fibre**

calcium. They also provide a source of fat if they are full fat types;

♦ meat, fish and alternatives – provide protein and minerals, especially iron, as well as vitamins; and

♦ foods containing fat and foods containing sugar – provide fat, particularly saturated fats, and also sugars.

Health problems related to a poor diet

Unfortunately the average diet eaten in this country is not reflective of that illustrated in the Balance of Good Health. Many people eat too much fat, especially excessive amounts of saturated fat, too little fruit and vegetables and not enough bread, other cereals and potatoes and far too much sugar, salt and alcohol.

There are major links between diet and health problems such as obesity, coronary heart disease and cancer.

MAIN GROUPS OF NUTRIENTS

The basic requirements of the body are often known as physiological requirements.

To live we need energy for body activities. This energy is derived from foods. Energy is measured in kilocalories (kcal), often referred to as calories and kilojoules (kJ).

Fluid is needed for survival and without adequate fluid we will only survive a few days at most.

There are five main groups of nutrients:
- ♦ protein;
- ♦ fat;
- ♦ carbohydrate;
- ♦ vitamins; and
- ♦ minerals.

Energy is provided by protein, fat and carbohydrate. Alcohol is not a necessary part of the diet but it also provides energy.

Vitamins and minerals are both vital for life but do not provide energy.

Foods are normally mixtures of a number of nutrients. Therefore a variety of different foods is required as part of a balanced diet. No one food is able to sustain adult life. Babies are able to thrive on breast milk for the first few months of life.

PHYSIOLOGICAL REQUIREMENTS

- • **Need fluid**

- • **Energy from foods**
  - • **Carbohydrate = 3.75 kcal per gram**
  - • **Protein = 4 kcal per gram**
  - • **Fat = 9 kcal per gram**
  - • **Alcohol = 7 kcal per gram**

  Energy also measured in joules:
  to convert kcal to kJ multiply by 4.184

- • **Vitamins**

- • **Minerals**

Macronutrients

Macronutrients are the nutrients required in large quantities. They therefore cover:

- protein;
- fat; and
- carbohydrate.

These are the nutrients which provide energy.

Micronutrients

Micronutrients are the group of nutrients which are required in small amounts and includes vitamins and minerals.

Trace elements or trace minerals are those minerals which are needed in minute amounts.

Chemistry of nutrients

Food and the nutrients they contain, like all substances, are composed of different chemical elements arranged in a variety of ways to form molecules. These molecules vary according to the elements they contain and how the different elements are linked together.

MICRONUTRIENTS	
Vitamins	**Minerals**
Thiamin	Calcium
Riboflavin	Phosphorus
Niacin	Iron
B_6	Magnesium
B_{12}	Sodium
Folate	Potassium
Vitamin C	Chloride
Vitamin A	Zinc
Vitamin D	Copper*
Vitamin E	Selenium*
Vitamin K	Iodine*
	Molybdenum*
	Cobalt*
	Manganese*
	Chromium*
	Fluoride*

* Trace elements

Units of measurements

Nutrition has a number of standard ways of measuring items.

Weights of foods and also of nutrients are measured in kilograms, grams, milligrams and micrograms.

Energy is measured in calories and joules. This measurement of energy can be either the energy obtained from macronutrients such as protein, fat, carbohydrate or alcohol or the energy expended in the Basal Metabolic Rate (BMR) or in activities such as walking.

Energy derived from foods is normally quoted as kcal per 100g of food. The energy for activities is normally quoted for the duration of time of the activity. Increasingly joules are being used to measure the energy of activity and foods.

UNITS
g = gram
mg = milligram (one thousandth of a gram)
µg = microgram (one millionth of a gram)
kg = kilogram (1000 grams)
kcal = kilocalorie (1000 calories)
kJ = kilojoule (1000 joules)
MJ = megajoule (million joules)
1 kcal = 4.184 kJ

Dietary reference values for food energy and nutrients for the UK

This report is a key document for nutritionists as it gives standards upon which to base the nutritional content of diets for groups such as those in schools and also for individuals. The report was produced by the Panel on Dietary Reference Values of the Committee of the Medical Aspects of Food Policy, which is often referred to as COMA, in 1991.

It contains a range of figures giving the various amounts of nutrients.

The figures in this report on dietary reference values provide information which has been derived from examination of numerous reports on nutrition on the amounts of energy and nutrients required by different age groups of the population and for males and females. The report also makes recommendations as to the proportions of energy that should be derived from different macronutrients.

DEFINITIONS
Dietary Reference Values for Food Energy and Nutrients for the United Kingdom (1991) COMA
• **DRV** **Dietary Reference Values includes EAR, LRNI & RNI**
• **EAR** **Estimated Average Requirement**
• **LRNI** **Lower Reference Nutrient Intake**
• **RNI** **Reference Nutrient Intake**

Proportions of energy which should be derived from different macronutrients

Health research shows that a greater proportion of our energy derived from food should be obtained from starchy carbohydrates such as bread, potatoes, rice, pasta and breakfast cereals.

Estimated Average Requirements

The report refers to the recommended amounts of energy as Estimated Average Requirements for energy, abbreviated as EAR.

As can be seen, the group with the highest requirements is males aged 15 to 18 years, as they normally are very active; they are also going through an active growth period.

It must however be remembered that these figures are an average and do not take into account individual variations. As they are average figures it will mean that a proportion of the population actually needs more than the figure quoted and other people will need less.

Also those with different needs such as very active sportspeople will have far higher energy requirements than those given in the chart of EAR.

ESTIMATED AVERAGE REQUIREMENTS FOR ENERGY

Age	Males kcal	Females kcal
0-3 months	545	515
4-6 months	690	645
7-9 months	825	765
10-12 months	920	865
1-3 years	1230	1165
4-6 years	1715	1545
7-10 years	1970	1740
11-14 years	2220	1845
15-18 years	2755	2110
19-50 years	2550	1940
51-59 years	2550	1900
60-64 years	2380	1900
65-74 years	2330	1900
75+ years	2100	1810

Pregnancy last third extra 200 kcal per day
Lactating 1st month extra 450 kcal per day
Lactating 2nd month extra 530 kcal per day
Lactating 3rd month extra 570 kcal per day
Lactating 4th-6th months extra 480 kcal per day

Reference Nutrient Intake (RNI)

The RNI is the term used to indicate the amount of protein, vitamins and minerals required for 97% of the population. The values for the figures are found in 'Dietary Reference Values for Food Energy and Nutrients for the UK' report of the Panel on Dietary Reference Values of the Committee of the Medical Aspects of Food Policy (1991).

Age range	Protein (g)	Calcium (mg)	Iron (mg)	Zinc (mg)	Vitamin A (μ)	Thiamin (mg)	Vitamin B6[a] (mg[a])	Folic acid (μg)	Vitamin C (mg)
0-3 months (formula fed)	12.5	525	1.7	4.0	350	0.2	0.2	50	25
4-6 months	12.7	525	4.3	4.0	350	0.2	0.2	50	25
7-9 months	13.7	525	7.8	5.0	350	0.2	0.3	50	25
10-12 months	14.9	525	7.8	5.0	350	0.3	0.4	50	25
1-3 years	14.5	350	6.9	5.0	400	0.5	0.7	70	30
4-6 years	19.7	450	6.1	6.5	500	0.7	0.9	100	30
7-10 years	28.3	550	8.7	7.0	500	0.7	1.0	150	30
Males									
11-14 years	42.1	1000	11.3	9.0	600	0.9	1.2	200	35
15-18 years	55.2	1000	11.3	9.5	700	1.1	1.5	200	40
19-50 years	55.5	700	8.7	9.5	700	1.0	1.4	200	40
50+ years	53.3	700	8.7	9.5	700	0.9	1.4	200	40
Females									
11-14 years	41.2	800	14.8	9.0	600	0.7	1.0	200	35
15-18 years	45.0	800	14.8	7.0	600	0.8	1.2	200	40
19-50 years	45.0	700	14.8	7.0	600	0.8	1.2	200	40
50+ years	46.5	700	8.7	7.0	600	0.8	1.2	200	40
Pregnant	+6.0				+100	+0.1[d]		+100	+10
Lactating:									
0-4 months	+11.0	+550		+6.0	+350	+0.2		+60	+30
over 4 months	+8.0	+550		+2.5	+350	+0.2		+60	+30

Lower Reference Nutrient Intake (LRNI)

The LRNI is the Lower Reference Nutrient Intake and is the amount of protein, vitamins and minerals required for only 3% of the population. Therefore this level meets the needs of only a few people.

Metabolism

The body is a complex living structure composed of billions of individual cells. The cells themselves consist of proteins and other nutrients bound together in certain ways that give each cell its own special function. Cells are grouped together into tissues and organs which perform specific functions. For example, the skin is the largest tissue in the body while the heart is the organ responsible for the circulation of blood.

Within the body chemical reactions are occurring all the time in cells, to enable them to carry out the processes of growth and repair needed for life. This complex collection of chemical reactions is called metabolism.

Energy is required for metabolism to occur. The energy is derived from foods such as carbohydrates, proteins and fats. Alcohol also provides energy.

Basal Metabolic Rate (BMR)

Energy is required for all of the metabolic actions to occur in the body. These processes include the basic ones required to keep us alive and include:

♦ breathing;
♦ heartbeat;
♦ maintenance of body temperature;
♦ brain activities;
♦ secretion of enzymes;
♦ production of hormones; and
♦ production of body tissues.

These activities are occurring continuously and as we are not aware of them they are referred to as involuntary activities. They all require energy and the amount of energy required is called the Basal Metabolic Rate, which is often abbreviated as the BMR.

The BMR is measured when someone is at complete rest both mentally and physically.

Energy requirements

Everyone needs energy from food to live. Energy is required for all of the vital functions of the body such as maintenance of the body temperature, breathing, digestion, blood circulation, hormone release and all of the other cellular activities that occur in the body. Additionally we need energy for all activities whether small ones such as reading or much more vigorous ones such as jogging. Energy is also needed for growth such as occurs in children and during pregnancy.

Energy is measured in both kilojoules and megajoules abbreviated as kJ and MJ respectively. Energy is also measured in kilocalories, abbreviated as kcal. The latter term is usually referred to as 'calories' and is familiar to anyone who has tried to control their calorie intake in an effort to lose weight.

Food labels are a source of information on the energy values of food; energy values are stated per 100g of food.

The whole area of energy contents of foods and meals can be one of confusion.

The simple way of converting energy in kilocalories to kilojoules (to give a good approximation) is to multiply by 4.2. Thus a food such as a digestive biscuit, which contains 70 kilocalories or calories, would provide about 294 kilojoules.

Energy is obtained from foods and is needed for the maintenance of life. This requirement includes the energy needed for the basal metabolic activities plus additional activities such as movements of the body, which require muscular activity. Such activities include reading, walking, running and driving.

Additional energy is required for growth and repair of body tissues. Growth occurs during childhood and adolescence. During pregnancy energy is needed for the growth of the foetus and also after the baby is born for the production of breast milk, during the period of lactation.

Energy is required for the repair of body tissues and anyone who has undergone an operation or accident will require additional energy for this process to occur.

The recommendations for the amount of energy needed for different individuals are called the Estimated Average Requirements (EAR).

EAR FOR TEENAGERS (15-18 YEARS)			
MALES		**FEMALES**	
MJ/day	Kcal/day	MJ/day	Kcal/day
11.51	2,755	8.83	2,110

Energy Balance

If more energy is consumed than is required, the body stores it up as fat. If insufficient energy is obtained from food then the body uses up stores of fat.

People may expend more energy than they are consuming from food due to exercising or healing occurring. Also maintaining the body temperature in very cold environments such as the Arctic can increase energy requirements.

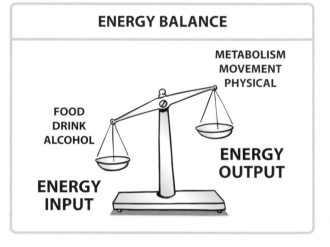

Foods providing energy

As described the macronutrients, protein, fat and carbohydrate all provide energy.

Protein provides 4 kilocalories of energy per gram, carbohydrate 3.75 kilocalories per gram and fat 9 kilocalories per gram.

As can be seen, fat provides a much more concentrated source of energy than protein or carbohydrate. Therefore fat is said to be an energy-dense food.

Percentage energy from fat in the diet

For a healthy diet we are recommended to limit the amount of fat, especially saturated fat, due to the links between fat and coronary heart disease. The recommended source of energy is from starchy carbohydrates such as bread, potatoes, pasta and rice.

It is recommended that the maximum percentage of the total amount of energy provided by fat in the diet is 35%. This is an important concept but is often misunderstood.

An example of the maximum amount of fat that should be taken by a 15-18 year old girl would be as follows:

♦ **the EAR is 2,110 kcal**

♦ **35% of this is 735**
   i.e. the maximum number of kcal which should be supplied by fat

♦ **to work out the actual number of grams of fat, 735 is divided by 9 (the amount of energy provided by 1g of fat), giving a figure of almost 82 grams of fat per day. This 82 grams of fat is derived from foods and beverages at three meals and also from snacks.**

The preferred source of energy for health is carbohydrates and around 50% of our energy should be taken from these. An example of the maximum amount of carbohydrate that should be taken by a 15-18 year old girl would be as follows:

- **the EAR is 2,110 kcal**

- **50% of this is 1055**
  i.e. the number of kcal which should be supplied by carbohydrate – preferably starchy ones

- **to work out the actual number of grams of carbohydrate, 1055 is divided by 3.75 (the amount of energy provided by 1g of carbohydrate), giving a figure of 281 grams of carbohydrate per day.**

This leaves 15% of the energy to be obtained from protein foods. To work this out as actual quantities of protein the following calculation is used:

- **the EAR is 2,110 kcal**

- **15% of this is 316**
  i.e. the number of kcal which should be supplied by proteins

- **to work out the actual number of grams of protein, 316 is divided by 4 (the amount of energy provided by 1g of protein), giving a figure of 79 grams of protein per day.**

Question to determine progress
Describe the Balance of Good Health and the five food groups it it contains. **See answer in the appendix.**

2 Factors affecting food intake and choice

There are a number of factors affecting food intake and choice. In underdeveloped countries poverty and limited access to food mean that food and fluid are taken to meet the basic physiological requirements of fluid and energy.

PHYSIOLOGICAL REQUIREMENTS

Physiology is the science that makes a study of the life processes and functions of living things. Therefore the physiological requirements are the basic nutritional requirements for life to occur.

The essential components of the diet to meet these physiological components are as follows.

PHYSIOLOGICAL REQUIREMENTS

- Fluid
- Energy from foods
  - **Carbohydrates = 3.75 kcal per gram**
  - **Protein = 4 kcal per gram**
  - **Fat = 9 kcal per gram**
  - **Alcohol = 7 kcal per gram**

Energy also measured in joules; to convert kcal to kJ multiply by 4.184

- Vitamins
- Minerals

Fluid

To live we need to take in fluid and nutrients. Without fluid we will not survive for more than 3 or 4 days, so a regular supply of fluid is essential.

Energy

Energy is required for all of the body activities to occur. These activities include the basal metabolic rate, which includes the maintenance of body temperature and growth and repair as well as movement.

Energy is provided by the nutrients carbohydrate, protein and fat. These are called macronutrients. Alcohol also provides energy.

The body is able to store a small amount of carbohydrate as glycogen in muscles and the liver to meet short-term energy needs. Larger amounts of energy are stored in the body as fat. Excessive deposits of body fat are harmful to health and can contribute to the development of coronary heart disease.

Substances for growth and repair

All cells of the body are continually being replaced and therefore substances for the growth and repair of body tissues are required. The main substances required for growth and repair are proteins and minerals.

Proteins are a key element in the diet needed for growth and the repair of body tissues. Protein is a key component of the skin, muscles, hair, nails, heart, lungs, intestines, blood and immune system. Growing children and teenagers need extra protein for growth of the body tissues to occur.

Minerals are also needed for growth and repair of body tissues. For example, calcium and phosphorus are vital for the correct development of bones, which make up the skeleton.

Iron is a key component of haemoglobin, which is the red colouring matter in the blood and which enables oxygen to be carried from the lungs to all parts of the body, where it is used in the energy release cycle of cells.

Zinc is a key component of the immune system of the body, which is the system that helps with fighting infections and diseases.

Substances which regulate the processes of energy production and growth

This group of nutrients includes the vitamins. For example, thiamin Vitamin B1 (one of the vitamin B group) is required for energy release from carbohydrates.

OTHER FACTORS AFFECTING FOOD INTAKE AND CHOICE

Hunger

Hunger is the sensation felt when the body needs food because the blood sugar level is low and the stomach is empty. The body responds to the thought of eating when hungry, by the mouth watering due to the production of saliva, and in the stomach hydrochloric acid is produced and in the intestines, digestive enzymes are produced. These responses prepare the body to cope with digesting the food eaten.

Appetite

The desire for food depends on aesthetics such as:

♦ appearance which includes the colour and way food is served;
♦ flavour;
♦ odour; and
♦ texture.

All of these aspects are important in affecting the enjoyment of food. Many of these factors are relevant to the individual, for example, one person may enjoy a cup of tea with sugar in it, while another person may be unable to drink it.

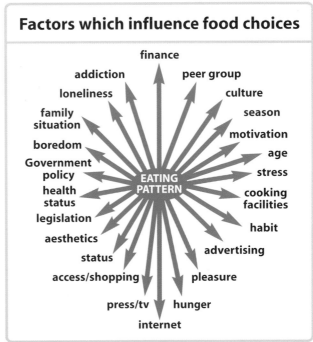

Factors which influence food choices

finance · addiction · peer group · loneliness · culture · family situation · season · boredom · motivation · Government policy · age · health status · stress · legislation · cooking facilities · aesthetics · habit · status · advertising · access/shopping · pleasure · press/tv · hunger · internet

EATING PATTERN

Age

Nutritional requirements vary according to age and gender. For example, the requirements for energy and protein in males are usually higher than those of females, due to the larger body size in males. Males also have proportionally more body muscle than women.

Teenagers aged 15-18 years old need more energy than adults due to their greater activity levels and growth still occurring.

Babies need proportionally more protein than adults. During lactation, when mothers are producing breast milk, more energy and protein are required.

Peer Group pressure

Teenagers are especially sensitive to peer group pressure, so that they may have to have similar food to their contemporaries, for example, brand leader crisps in their lunch boxes.

Cultural and social influences

Nowadays Britain is a diverse multicultural society. Some areas and communities may have numerous cultural groups whilst others may have just one main group and yet others may have a totally indigenous group wanting traditional British fare or rather a range of international fare.

This means there are tremendous variations in the acceptability of different foods as part of meals. What is an accepted food by one group may not be acceptable to another group of the same faith. Sometimes even within a household some members of a family who were born in this country may accept a wider variety of foods than older siblings who were born abroad. Sometimes whilst certain foods are not eaten at home in deference to more traditional dietary practices by grandparents, away from home the same foods are enjoyed.

Cultural groups include:

♦   those from the Jewish community;
♦   Muslim groups; and
♦   Afro-Caribbean groups.

There is a range of different types of vegetarians, who follow the diet for different reasons, which may be ethical, religious or even because of individual likes and dislikes. Lacto-ovo vegetarians take no animal foods such as meat or fish. They do take milk and eggs. Most people who say they are vegetarian belong to this group. Demi-vegetarians are those who take small amounts of fish and poultry as well as milk and eggs. Vegans take no food of animal origins, so they do not eat milk or eggs.

Food availability and seasonal variation

Because of the availability of imported food, the effect of seasons on food availability is not as apparent as it was in the past. However, in general people tend to enjoy salads in summer and soups or casseroles in cold winter weather.

Some people are becoming more interested in local food with farmers' markets.

Menus in restaurants, schools and hospitals have local food featuring in them now. The term 'provenance of food' means that one knows where food is derived from.

Finance

Finance is an important aspect of food choice. For those with not much money, for example, those on a pension or those on benefits, the cost of food can be a predominant factor.

Nowadays we tend to spend less on food as a percentage of our total income, as food has become relatively inexpensive.

Also today on average we tend to eat out three times per week. This includes meals in fast food restaurants and in workplace canteens.

Motivation
Not bothering to cook or shop affects those on their own, especially elderly people.

Stress
Stress and the effect of this may either increase the appetite with comfort eating or reduce the appetite.

Boredom
People may eat because they are bored. Also people may drink alcohol to cheer themselves up.

Family situations
The family situation in which people live may have a significant effect on what is eaten, for example, with celebration meals or regular meals at the table. Other families may eat meals mainly on their laps in front of the TV.

Loneliness
Loneliness and depression may mean people eat snacks rather than cook and eat proper meals.

Cooking facilities
For caterers, the menus will be affected by the catering equipment that is available to prepare and store food.

For families and those living on their own, storage and cooking facilities play a large part in the food that is eaten. For example, someone living in a bed-sitter is unlikely to have full cooking and storage facilities.

Habit
Habits regarding meals and food play an important factor in what people eat. For example, if one is brought up to have breakfast it is difficult to break this habit in later life. If meals are eaten at the table then this habit tends to persist.

Advertising
Advertisements, whether on TV, in the press or in magazines, both encourage and inform people about products. Children may often be susceptible to putting pressure on parents to buy products in response to seeing advertisements. The Advertising Standards Authority (ASA) assists in ensuring that advertisements are not misleading.

Many other aspects of the media also have an effect on food choice with images of supermodels and their slender shape encouraging slimming. Also images of activity and fitness may encourage an interest in healthy eating.

Pleasure
Food and the flavour of it as well as the environment of a mealtime encourage one to eat. Sitting with a group of friends eating a leisurely meal may encourage one to eat more rather than when one is rushed.

Access to food

The ease of obtaining food will have a major effect on what people eat. How near supermarkets and shops are has an impact on what people eat. Many supermarkets are built on out-of-town estates, so people need cars to shop in them. Some people such as the elderly and disabled may not be able to drive. Even if there is public transport, carrying sufficient food for a family may be difficult.

Some smaller shops may not have a good range of foods, especially fruit and vegetables. Also food may be more expensive.

Status

Certain foods are perceived to be more appropriate to those with a higher status such as regular meals out in expensive restaurants. Such regular eating out may contribute to a high fat intake.

Legislation

Laws on food labelling such as those on food hygiene (which is not part of this book) and other legislation have an effect on diet.

Such legislation includes adding vitamins such as thiamin (vitamin B1), iron, calcium carbonate and niacin (one of the B vitamins) to white flour. Vitamins A and D are added to margarines. Iodine is added to iodised table salt

School meals have to meet certain nutritional standards.

In some local areas fluoride is added to the water supply. This is allowed in some areas at a level of 1ppm of fluoride to water.

Government Policy

The Food Standards Agency produces policies on food and health. It is a Non-Governmental Department responsible for providing advice and information to the public and government on food safety, nutrition and diet. The Food Standards Agency aims to put the consumer first and to be open and accessible and be an independent voice.

Other government departments such as the Department of Health and Department for Environment Farming and Rural Affairs also produce information and policies on food and nutrition.

Addiction

Addictions to food and beverages can occur. The obvious one is alcohol, which can be a major source of calories and can contribute to obesity, especially what is called central obesity in men. In this type of obesity the weight is distributed mainly around the stomach area of the body.

Some people can be addicted to caffeine and get withdrawal headaches when they cease taking it. Chocolate contains caffeine as well as a number of other substances and can be difficult for some people to exclude from their diet.

Internet

The internet provides information on food and diet such as information on diabetes. Also enables people to order shopping on-line.

Health status

People who are ill may not eat well due to a loss of appetite. Any individual who has a health problem requiring a special diet, e.g. for diabetes or cholesterol lowering diet will require to modify their intake. For example, those requiring a diet for diabetes will need to avoid adding sugar to drinks and cereals and those requiring a cholesterol lowering diet will require a diet low in saturated fat.

Anyone with a food allergy will need to avoid certain foods, for example, those with a milk allergy will need to avoid any foods where milk is an ingredient.

Effect of diet and health

Numerous medical and consumer reports from such organisations as the Committee of Medical Aspects of Food Policy, the World Health Organisation (WHO), the Food Standards Agency and other expert reports make various recommendations on diet and health.

In general these recommendations are to eat less saturated fat, to avoid becoming overweight, to take plenty of fruit and vegetables and take plenty of starchy carbohydrate.

Many people are influenced by these reports. The reports are often covered in articles in magazines and newspapers as well as being widely advocated by health professionals.

Some people are also advised by doctors and dietitians to alter their diet for individual health reasons such as being diagnosed with a milk intolerance. Such a person will need to avoid milk and products containing milk, which could have an effect on the family's diet.

Question to determine progress

Detail the factors affecting the food choice of:

♦ a teenage boy at school;
♦ an elderly lady living on her own in the country; and
♦ a family of four living in high rise accommodation with no car, the parents both work long hours and the children are both at secondary school.

See answer in the appendix.

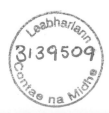

3 Macronutrients

Macronutrients are the nutrients required in large quantities which provide energy, and comprise:

◆   protein which provides 4 kcal energy per gram;
◆   fat which provides 9 kcal energy per gram; and
◆   carbohydrate which provides 3.75 kcal energy per gram.

PROTEINS

Humans need a regular supply of protein in their diet. The main sources of proteins are meats, offal, poultry, fish, eggs, cheese, milk and yoghurts. For vegetarians and vegans, nuts and pulses such as peas, beans and lentils all provide protein.

Often there can be confusion as to which foods supply proteins and some may consider that foods such as rice (which contains only a small amount of protein) are a good source of protein. This confusion is not surprising as it is noted that even some authors of books on nutrition wrongly quote sources of protein.

Chemical elements which comprise proteins

The key chemical element that is found in amino acids, which make up proteins, is nitrogen. Proteins also contain carbon, hydrogen and oxygen. Some amino acids contain phosphorus and others contain sulphur.

The element that is unique to all proteins is nitrogen.

The main sources of proteins are meats, offal, poultry, fish, eggs, cheese, milk and yoghurts

For vegetarians and vegans, nuts and pulses such as peas, beans and lentils all provide protein

Where proteins are found in the human body

The average adult human weighing about 70kg contains about 11kg of protein. Protein is a major component of the cells which make up all organs of the body. About 43% of body proteins are found in the muscle tissues, 21% in the skin, 19% in the blood and 5% in the liver. The brain, kidneys, hair, nails and other vital organs all also contain protein. Proteins are also key components of hormones and enzymes such as digestive enzymes.

Part of the immune system (the system responsible for helping the body to fight off infections and illnesses) is made up of proteins.

These tissue proteins of the body are continually being broken down and reformed during the process of protein turnover. Therefore humans need a regular supply of protein in their diet.

Requirements for protein

Requirements for protein for the general population, which would meet the needs of 97% of individuals, are specified as Reference Nutrient Intakes.

The reference nutrient intake for protein is 55.5g per day in adult males aged 19-50 years and 55.3g in those males over 50 years of age. The reference nutrient intake for protein is 45.0g per day in adult females aged 19-50 years and 46.5g in those females over 50 years of age. During pregnancy an extra 6.0g of protein per day is required. In the first four months of breast-feeding this requirement increases to 11g of protein per day.

In general this recommendation is based on a figure of 0.75g/protein per kg/body weight per day. Some individuals such as those with problems with wounds and burns may need far greater quantities than this in their diet.

Increased requirements for protein during illnesses

During periods of injury or infection the situation can occur where more body tissue proteins are lost than reformed. During this process the person is said to be in negative nitrogen balance.

If the situation continues without replacement of the body proteins by dietary means, such as can occur during starvation, then further protein breakdown occurs as the body uses protein as a source of energy. This is referred to as protein energy malnutrition and has been found to a moderate extent in surgical, general and orthopaedic patients. However, in geriatric and respiratory medicine, severe protein energy malnutrition has been found.

Such a situation can occur in a sick individual who for various reasons is unable to eat.

As already described, protein is required for the formation of body tissues such as muscle and skin. Therefore during the process of wound healing such as occurs post-operatively and after traumas such as road traffic accidents or severe burns, proteins need to be supplied by the diet to enable the body to synthesise tissues such as connective tissue.

Large open wounds can also discharge protein and a large open wound can lose 90-100g of protein per day.

For the patients who have not undergone surgery, trauma or who are only in hospital for a few days, excessive amounts of protein are not recommended due to effects on the filtration rate of the kidney. Some patients may have kidney problems and thus need a measured amount of protein per day. The guidelines on nutrition for hospital catering used to recommend that each main meal supplied 18g of protein.

Amino acids

Proteins are made up of chains of amino acids. Amino acids are the building blocks from which proteins are made. Some of these amino acids are called indispensible or essential amino acids as they cannot be made in the body but must be supplied by the diet. There are eight such amino acids in adults and nine in children.

Foods containing all of the essential amino acids are ones such as meat, offal, fish, milk, eggs and cheese. Some vegetable-based foods such as pulses may have a limited content of

EIGHT **ESSENTIAL AMINO ACIDS**

Eight essential amino acids for adults

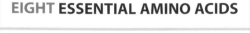

* **Isoleucine**

* **Phenylalanine**

* **Leucine**

* **Threonine**

* **Lysine**

* **Tryptophan**

* **Methionine**

* **Valine**

Histidine is indispensable for infants because of their rapid growth rate

one of the essential amino acids and therefore this needs to be supplied by other food in the diet which contain the amino acid in the limited quantity.

The remaining amino acids are called non-essential amino acids.

THE REMAINING AMINO ACIDS

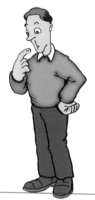

* **Alanine**
* **Glutamine**
* **Arginine**
* **Glycine**
* **Aspartic acid**
* **Asparagine**
* **Cysteine**
* **Glutamic acid**
* **Proline**
* **Serine**
* **Tyrosine**

Metabolic disorders

Some people can suffer from metabolic problems such as phenylketonuria, where the amount of a specific amino acid in the diet needs to be carefully controlled.

Sources of protein

The major sources of protein in the diet are meat, eggs, fish, cheese and pulses. These foods contain around 20g of protein per 100g of food. Potatoes, rice, fruit and green vegetables are all known to contain relatively low levels of protein.

Milk contains relatively low levels of protein. Because of the amounts of milk taken each day in drinks such as teas and coffees as well as its use in dishes such as white sauces, custards and mousses, it can provide a good contribution to protein intake.

Increasing the amount of protein in dishes

The amount of protein in a dish can be easily increased by adding dried skimmed milk powder to milk itself for use on cereals and in teas and coffees. Dried skimmed milk powder can be added to mashed potatoes, sauces, puddings and pork, fish and chicken dishes where a white sauce is used.

Cheese toppings can be added to potato dishes and extra snacks of cheese and biscuits given between meals will also help to improve a patient's protein intake. Meat or chicken can be puréed and added to soups to provide additional protein.

THE PERCENTAGE OF PROTEIN IN VARIOUS FOODS

FOOD	GRAMS OF PROTEIN PER 100g OF FOOD
Cod, frozen, raw	16.7
Salmon raw	20.2
Lamb, average, extra trimmed lean, raw	20.0
Pork, average, trimmed lean, raw	21.8
Beef, average, extra trimmed lean, raw	21.6
Chicken, meat, average, raw	23.3
Cashew nuts	17.7
Lentils, red, dried, raw, uncooked	23.8
Eggs, raw	12.5
Cheese cheddar, average	25.5
Semi-skimmed milk, pasteurised, average	3.3
Dried skimmed milk	36.1
White rice raw, uncooked	6.5
White bread	8.4
Macaroni raw, uncooked	12.0
Cauliflower, raw	3.6
New potatoes, average, raw	1.7
Apples, eating, raw	0.4

FATS

There are various types of fat, or lipids as they may sometimes be called. Whether saturated, monounsaturated or polyunsaturated, all fats provide 9kcal per gram and are thus equal as regards a source of energy. Too much energy in the diet can contribute to weight gain. We should take no more than 35% of the energy from fat in the diet.

Saturated fats are derived from sources such as full cream milks, full fat cheese, lard, butter, the fat found on meat and other fatty foods such as pastry.

Polyunsaturated fats are those derived from oils such as soya, corn, fish and soya oils. These oils are thought to be beneficial but still provide a source of calories.

Monounsaturated fats such as are found in olive oil are thought to be beneficial to the heart.

Chemical elements which comprise fats and the chemical structure of fats

Fats are made up of fatty acids; which are composed of carbon, hydrogen and oxygen. Fatty acids usually consist of a glycerol molecule and three fatty acids linked to it. The fatty acids can be either saturated or unsaturated.

The carbon atoms in the fatty acids are linked together by bonds. These bonds can be double bonds or single bonds. The double bonds are not completely saturated with hydrogen atoms and are therefore termed unsaturated.

> **FATS (LIPIDS)**
>
> • **Fatty acids**
>
> • **Contain**
>   • **Carbon**
>   • **Hydrogen**
>   • **Oxygen**
>
> • **Double bonds present in unsaturated fats**
>   • **One in monounsaturated fats**
>   • **Two or more in polyunsaturated fats**

EXAMPLE OF AN UNSATURATED FATTY ACID

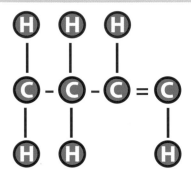

H represents hydrogen molecules
C represents carbon molecules
= represents a double bond
– represents a single bond
As can be seen more hydrogen molecules could be accepted

EXAMPLE OF A SATURATED FATTY ACID

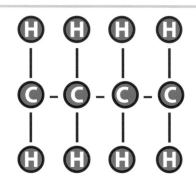

H represents hydrogen molecules
C represents carbon molecules
– represents a single bond

SATURATED FATS

Saturated fats are found in:

- **Butter**
- **Hard cheese**
- **Lard**
- **Dripping**
- **Coconut oil**
- **Palm oil**

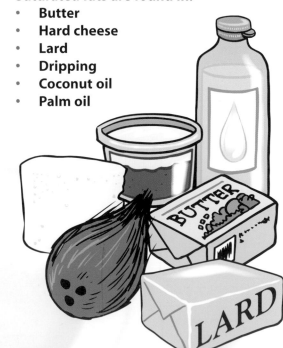

Unsaturated bonds mean that more hydrogen molecules could be accepted.

Saturated fats

In saturated fats all of the carbon atoms are saturated and only single bonds are present. An example of a saturated fatty acid is butyric acid found in butter.

Other saturated fats are found in butter, hard cheese, lard, dripping, coconut oil and palm oil. Foods containing any of these fats will also have a high proportion of saturated fat in them.

Monounsaturated fats

In monounsaturated fats there is a double bond between two of the carbon atoms in the fatty acid. Examples of monounsaturated fatty acids are oleic acid found in olive oil and rapeseed oil.

Monounsaturated fats are more beneficial to health as they help to lower the level of low-density lipoprotein cholesterol (LDL) but do not lower the level of high-density lipoprotein cholesterol (HDL), which is the beneficial type of cholesterol.

Monounsaturated fats are linked with a healthy diet and a reduced rate of coronary heart disease such as is found in Mediterranean areas.

Polyunsaturated fats

In polyunsaturated fats there are two or more double bonds between the carbon atoms. Examples of polyunsaturated fatty acids are linoleic and linolenic acids found in plant oils.

Polyunsaturated spreads are specially manufactured so as to retain a proportion of the polyunsaturated fatty acids.

Polyunsaturated fats are beneficial to health like monounsaturated as they lower the level of low-density lipoprotein cholesterol (LDL) but do

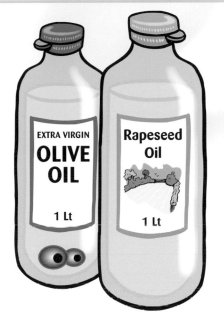

UNSATURATED FATS
(MONOUNSATURATED)

EXTRA VIRGIN
OLIVE OIL
1 Lt

Rapeseed Oil
1 Lt

Monounsaturated fats are found in:
- Olive oil
- Rapeseed oil
- Walnut oil
- Avocado

Some margarines and spreads are made from monounsaturated fats

UNSATURATED FATS
(POLYUNSATURATED)

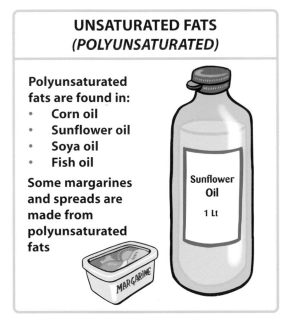

Polyunsaturated fats are found in:
- Corn oil
- Sunflower oil
- Soya oil
- Fish oil

Some margarines and spreads are made from polyunsaturated fats

Sunflower Oil
1 Lt

not lower the level of high-density lipoprotein cholesterol (HDL), which is the beneficial type of cholesterol. Therefore they are linked with the prevention of coronary heart disease.

Essential fatty acids

Certain polyunsaturated fatty acids are called essential as they cannot be made by the body and therefore must be provided by the diet. Examples are linoleic and alpha linoleic acid. Both of these fatty acids are essential for cell membranes in the body.

AMOUNTS OF FAT PER 100g FOOD

	g/100g food	Saturated	Monosaturated	Polyunsaturated
Butter	82.2	72	25	3
Margarine, soft	80.0	35	47	18
Margarine, polyunsaturated	68.5	25	23	52
Rapeseed oil	99.9	7	62	31
Sunflower oil	99.9	13	21	66
Milk, whole cows'	4.0	71	26	3
Eggs	11.2	35	47	18
Cheese, Cheddar	32.7	71	26	3
Beef, mince	15.7	51	47	2
Pork, chops	15.7	38	44	18
Biscuits, chocolate chip	22.9	49	39	12
Potato crisps	11.0	68	30	2
Peanuts	46.0	20	50	30

Omega-3 and Omega-6 fatty acids

Fatty acids can be classified according to the position of the double bond on the chain of carbon atoms.

Omega-3 fatty acids can help prevent blood clotting so they are particularly helpful in preventing coronary heart disease. They are also helpful in preventing inflammation and thus may be beneficial in joint diseases.

Sources of omega-3 fatty acids are fish oils, particularly those from oily fish.

Omega-6 fatty acids can help prevent coronary heart disease as they reduce levels of LDL cholesterol.

Sources of omega-6 fatty acids are sunflower oil, corn oil and soya oils.

Trans and cis fatty acids

The double bonds found in fatty acids can be orientated as to be in a cis or trans position.

Most natural fats contain cis double bonds. However, in manufacturing margarines the polyunsaturated fats are hydrogenated and more trans-fatty acid bonds are formed.

UNSATURATED FATS (OMEGA-3)

Omega-3 fats are a particular type of polyunsaturated fat. They can help prevent blood clotting & help reduce triglyceride levels.

Omega-3 fats are found in:
- Fish oil

Oily fish such as herring, kippers, mackerel, pilchards, sardines, salmon, trout and anchovies

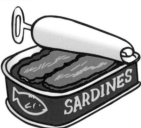

Our bodies can also make omega-3 fats from rapeseed oil, and from the oil in walnuts and soya

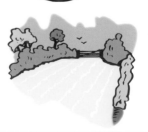

These trans-fatty acids are considered to be similar to saturated fats in their effect on health and are linked with coronary heart disease. We are recommended to have no more than 2% of our dietary energy from trans-fatty acids.

Cholesterol

Cholesterol is a sticky wax-like substance. It is essential to life and is:
   ◆   a component of cell walls;
   ◆   needed for the synthesis of bile salts necessary for fat digestion;
   ◆   required for the production of steroid hormones; and
   ◆   needed to manufacture vitamin D in the body.

Cholesterol circulates in the blood and a measurement of it indicates a risk of coronary heart disease. There are 2 types of cholesterol, normally:
   ◆   low-density lipoprotein cholesterol (LDL) the more harmful type of cholesterol; and
   ◆   high-density lipoprotein cholesterol (HDL) which is the beneficial cholesterol or protective type of cholesterol.

Besides being eaten in certain foods in the diet, cholesterol is also produced by the liver. LDL cholesterol is considered to be undesirable as it can be deposited in artery walls, thus contributing to coronary heart disease. A high proportion of saturated fat in the diet predisposes the production of LDL cholesterol, whereas both polyunsaturated fats and monosaturated fats can help to lower the LDL cholesterol without lowering the HDL cholesterol.

Cholesterol is found in relatively few foods. Food sources of cholesterol are egg yolks, liver and shellfish. We are recommended to have no more than 11% of the energy in our diet from saturated fat.

Triglycerides

These are sticky substances found in the blood. High levels are undesirable and contribute to coronary heart disease. High levels are related to excess saturated fat, alcohol, sugar and obesity.

Functions of fat in the body

A certain amount of fat is needed in the diet to provide the essential fatty acids, which are vital in the production of cell membranes in the body.

The fat-soluble vitamins A, D, E and K are found alongside fats in the diet.

Fat is a source of energy in the diet and as it provides 9kcal per gram fats, it is the most concentrated form of energy in the diet (protein provides 4kcal per gram and carbohydrate 3.75kcal per gram).

Adipose tissue

If we take in too much energy from food in our diet the body stores this up as fat in adipose tissue. This tissue is found around the vital organs like the lungs, heart, kidneys and intestines. There it offers some cushioning effect and protection.

Adipose tissue is found below the skin and excessive quantities can be deposited in the abdominal area. The excessive deposition of body fat is termed obesity.

Women naturally have a greater proportion of body fat than men, with approximately 25% of the body comprising of fat compared with 14% in men. Women store this fat mainly on breasts, hips and thighs, giving the characteristic female shape.

The percentage of fat on a woman's body is related to her ability to conceive. Women who are underweight and have only 10-15% body fat stop having monthly periods (amenorrhoea) and compromise their ability to conceive. Excessive amounts of body fat also reduce the ability to conceive.

Health aspects of fat

In the UK both men and women have an increased risk of coronary heart disease. Both obesity and raised cholesterol levels can contribute to the development of coronary heart disease.

High levels of saturated fat in a person's diet can contribute to both the development of raised cholesterol levels and obesity with a resultant increased risk of coronary heart disease.

Excessive amounts of fat in the diet can obviously lead to obesity and many diets for weight loss (slimming diets) are based on low fat foods. High fat foods are higher in the energy content than the equivalent quantity of low fat foods.

Breast cancer has also been linked with excessive quantities of fat in the diet.

Food sources of fat

Foods usually contain a mixture of different types of fat. For example, 100g of beef, average trimmed lean raw, contains 5.1g of fat; 100g of pork, average trimmed lean raw, contains 4.0g of fat; and 100 g of lamb, average trimmed raw, contains 8.3g of fat. Many of the packs of meat found are much lower than this with joints of fully trimmed pork containing less than 2% fat.

About half of the fat found in red meat is in the unsaturated form, which is believed to be healthier. Surveys show that meat is a major contributor of monounsaturated fat in the diet. Monounsaturated fats are the type found in olive oil. Useful amounts of polyunsaturated fatty acids are found in red meat. Polyunsaturated fat is associated with a lower risk of heart disease.

Attention has focused on the omega-3 fatty acids as evidence suggests they are beneficial in conditions such as rheumatoid arthritis. While these fatty acids are particularly abundant in oily fish, however, meat also provides them. In Britain we get approximately 20% of our intake from meat.

VISIBLE AND INVISIBLE FATS

Visible fats are those which are easily seen as fat. This group includes:

♦ butter;
♦ lard;
♦ oil;
♦ fat on meat;
♦ margarine;
♦ low fat spreads (these contain 25-70% fat);
♦ polyunsaturated spread;
♦ suet; and
♦ cream.

Invisible fats are those which are hidden in foods. This group includes:

♦ nuts;
♦ seeds;
♦ full fat milk (silver top);
♦ egg yolk;
♦ cheese - even low fat Cheddar cheese contains approximately 17% fat;
♦ lean meat;
♦ oily fish;
♦ pastry;
♦ cakes;
♦ biscuits;
♦ sauces;
♦ cheese spread;
♦ ice cream;
♦ fried foods;
♦ croquettes;
♦ chips (deep fried);
♦ samosas; and
♦ crisps.

As can be seen there is an extensive list of foods containing invisible fat.

Foods containing low levels of fat

We are encouraged to reduce the level of fat in our diet. Foods which are low in fat are:

♦ all types of fruit and vegetables, with the exception of olives and avocados;
♦ bread, potatoes, pasta, rice, breakfast cereals;
♦ lean red meat (pork, beef and lamb);
♦ poultry with no skin;
♦ rabbit and game;
♦ skimmed milk;
♦ cottage cheese; and
♦ low fat yoghurts.

Low-fat cooking methods

If low-fat foods are fried, such as potatoes made into chips, then this will add extra fat. Therefore it is advocated that low-fat cooking methods are used both within the home and in catering.

Cooking methods which provide less fat are:

♦ steaming;
♦ poaching;
♦ braising;
♦ casseroling;
♦ baking;
♦ simmering;
♦ grilling;

♦ boiling;

♦ barbecuing;

♦ stewing; and

♦ dry frying without fat.

If frying is used for foods it is better to fry items such as plain cuts of meat as these will absorb less fat than any foods which have breadcrumb or batter coatings.

CARBOHYDRATES

There are two main types of carbohydrates, sugary ones and starchy ones. Sugary ones include sugar, jams, sugary soft drinks, sweets, cakes, honeys, sweet biscuits and desserts. Sugary carbohydrates have been strongly linked with dental decay.

Starchy carbohydrates include bread, potatoes, pasta, breakfast cereals, rice and couscous.

Both types of carbohydrates provide the same amount of energy (3.75 kcal per g). Carbohydrates provide less than half the amount of energy provided by fat, gram for gram.

The preferred source of energy for health is starchy carbohydrates and most of the energy in the diet should be derived from starchy carbohydrates. Sugar is not required for energy.

Most of the carbohydrate in our diet comes from plants, for example, wheat, rice and oats, but some comes from milk and milk products.

Dietary fibre or non-starch polysaccharide (NSP) is also a form of carbohydrate. However, this type of carbohydrate cannot be digested by the body.

Chemical elements which comprise carbohydrates

Although there are several types of carbohydrate, they all contain the elements carbon, hydrogen and oxygen.

Plants produce carbohydrates by the process of photosynthesis, which uses energy from sunlight to produce carbohydrate from carbon dioxide and water.

CARBOHYDRATES

- Contain
  - **Carbon**
  - **Hydrogen**
  - **Oxygen**

- Sugars
  - **Monosaccharides (simple sugars)**
    e.g. glucose, fructose, galactose
  - **Disaccharides (two monosaccharides)**
    e.g. sucrose, maltose, lactose

- Starches (polysaccharides)
  - **amylose – straight chains**
  - **amylopectins – branch chains**
  - **glycogen**

- Non-starch polysaccharides (NSP)
  - **fibres**
  - **cellulose, pectins, lignins**

- Extrinsic sugars
  - **non-milk extrinsic sugar**

Sugars

Sugars consist of both monosaccharides (sometimes called simple sugars) and disaccharides. Both types of sugar are soluble in water and sweet to the taste.

There are three main monosaccharides:

1. Fructose or fruit sugar is found in fruits and honey.

2. Galactose is found as a component of the sugar found in milk.
3. Glucose is the main sugar found in starches. Glucose is also the form of carbohydrate that the body uses for energy, and is found circulating in the blood.

Disaccharides are sometimes called double sugars as they consist of two monosaccharides joined together. There are three disaccharides:

1. Sucrose consists of one unit of glucose joined to one unit of fructose. Sucrose is commonly seen as table sugar and is used in cookery. Most sucrose is obtained from sugar beet which is grown in this country in East Anglia, or from sugar cane grown in tropical countries.
2. Lactose consists of one unit of glucose joined to one unit of galactose. Lactose is found in milk, both from animals and in human breast milk.
3. Maltose consists of two units of glucose joined to each other. It is called malt sugar and is found in cereals.

Starches (polysaccharides)

'Poly' means many and starches are made up of many units of glucose joined together. If the glucose units are joined together in a straight chain this is amylose. When the glucose units are joined together in a branched chain it is called amylopectin.

During the process of digestion, starches are broken down to their component glucose units.

Glycogen

This is formed by the body in humans and animals from glucose. It is a form of polysaccharide, which is stored in small amounts in the liver and muscles to provide a temporary store of glucose for energy.

Non-starch polysaccharide (NSP)

We are all encouraged to take plenty of dietary fibre, or non-starch polysaccharide (NSP) as it is correctly called. Dietary fibre used to be called roughage. This has a protective effect on the bowel and helps to prevent constipation, diverticular disease, haemorrhoids and bowel cancer. We are advised to take about 18g of dietary fibre each day but on average we take only 12g.

Fibre is derived from plants and consists of such substances as cellulose, lignins and other fibres, which give structure to the plant. In these fibres the glucose units are joined in such a way as to make them unable to be attacked by digestive enzymes. Therefore NSP passes through the digestive tract and adds bulk to the diet.

There are 2 types of dietary fibre or NSP

◆   Soluble fibre: this has a beneficial effect on blood cholesterol and blood sugar levels. Soluble fibre is also helpful for bowel health. A number of people have problems such as diabetes with the associated raised blood sugar levels while others have heart disease and raised cholesterol levels. Therefore the inclusion of more soluble fibre in the diet can be of great benefit.
    Soluble fibre is found in all types of fruit and vegetables. Fruit juice does not contain much fibre as this is left with the fruit residue as the juice is extracted. Such new products as fruit smoothies have more fibre in them than do the juices. Pulses

are particularly rich in soluble fibre. Dried fruits are also good sources of soluble fibre.

♦ Insoluble fibre is found in wholewheat products such as wholemeal bread and wholewheat breakfast cereals. This is beneficial to bowel health.

Intrinsic and extrinsic sugars

Intrinsic sugars are those contained in the structure of foods such as sugars in fruits. Extrinsic sugars are those added in manufacturing foods such as in cakes.

It is recommended that only 10% of our energy is derived from extrinsic sugars.

Refined and unrefined carbohydrates

Refined carbohydrates are those which have undergone more processing and removal of NSP. Examples of these are white flour and white rice.

Unrefined carbohydrates are those which have been processed to a lesser extent such as wholemeal flour and brown rice.

Glycaemic Index (GI)

The GI is a measure of how carbohydrate foods are broken down by the body and therefore how fast they cause a rise in blood sugar level.

Foods with a low GI cause a slow rise in blood sugar and are considered to be more filling. Such foods with a low GI are oats, pulses and peanuts.

Carbohydrate requirements

At least half of the energy in our diets should come from carbohydrate, and mostly from starch. In the UK the average total carbohydrate intake per person per day is about 218g.

For sportspeople the proportion of energy from carbohydrate may be increased further to provide between 60 and 70% of energy. To achieve this, meals and snacks need to be high in carbohydrate.

Sources of carbohydrate

Different foods contain different amounts of carbohydrate.

♦ sugars are naturally found in milk, honey and fruit but are also added to many prepared foods (for example, biscuits, puddings, sweets and soft drinks); and

---

DIETARY FIBRE (NON-STARCH POLYSACCHARIDE)

- **2 types**
- **Soluble fibre**
  oats, lentils, peas, dried beans, fruit and vegetables

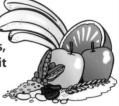

- **Insoluble fibre**
  wholemeal bread, brown pasta, bran-based cereals e.g. branflakes

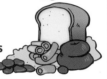

CARBOHYDRATE

- **2 main types of carbohydrate**
  - **sugars - refined**
  - **starch - refined and unrefined**
    - **both provide the same amount of energy**

- **Sources of starch include breakfast cereals and cereal foods (e.g. wheat, rice, maize, oats, rye, barley), roots and tubers (e.g. yams, cassava, potatoes, root vegetables), pulses and some fruit**

- **Sugars naturally found in milk, honey and fruit**

- **Added to many prepared foods (e.g. biscuits, puddings, sweets and soft drinks)**

◆　sources of starch include breakfast cereals and cereal foods (for example, wheat, rice, maize, cassava, oats, rye, barley), roots and tubers (for example, yams, potatoes, root vegetables), pulses and some fruit.

Sugar and dental decay

Frequent consumption of added sugars has been linked to dental decay, particularly where dental hygiene is poor.

Ways of boosting the amount of carbohydrate in the diet

Starchy carbohydrates have minimum amounts of fat in them and thus can be used to enhance the amount of energy derived from carbohydrate. Of particular use can be the inclusion of soluble fibre found in oats, pulses (for example, lentils, beans, peas and chickpeas), and also fruit and vegetables of all types.

◆　bread of various types can be taken as an accompaniment to meals. Pitta bread and wraps can be filled and provided as hand-held snacks, which are popular. Bread-based pizzas are tasty but ensure only a tiny amount of cheese is used. Garlic bread made with a minimum of butter can be served with pasta or pizzas. Naan breads can be served with curries or stir-fries;

◆　noodles can form a basis of stir-fries made with a minimum amount of fat;

◆　pasta can be served as an accompaniment such as spaghetti with Bolognese sauce, or as part of a macaroni and tuna bake;

◆　couscous can be used in wraps and as accompaniments to tagines;

◆　oats can be used to thicken dishes like casseroles. A handful of oats can be added to crumbles and biscuits to give an extra crunch to the dish. Oat bran can also be added to dishes;

◆　rice of all types can be served as part of a dish such as a risotto or accompanying a dish. A variety of rice salads can be made. It can also form the basis of puddings, for example, rice pudding made with skimmed milk and a sweetener; and

◆　potatoes can be served as part of a dish such as shepherd's pie, curries and salads or as accompaniments. Potatoes can be mashed, baked, boiled, roast or chipped. To limit the amount of fat absorbed, use large pieces of potato when making chips or potato wedges. Potato chips can be oven-baked rather than deep-fried. Roast potatoes can be made by spraying or brushing with oil rather than immersing in fat.

Question to determine progress

Write notes on proteins. **See answer in the appendix.**

4 Micronutrients

Micronutrients are vitamins and minerals which are needed in the diet in small amounts, hence the name 'micro' nutrients. Some of the minerals are needed in very small amounts and are called trace elements or trace minerals.

The quantities of vitamins and minerals recommended to be consumed in the diet for individuals of different age and gender are found in the report Dietary Reference Values for Food Energy and Nutrients for the UK produced by COMA in 1991.

VITAMINS

Vitamins are essential to life (the name vitamin is derived from the word 'vital'). They are needed in only small amounts and are required for various metabolic functions in the body.

There are two major types of vitamins: fat-soluble and water-soluble vitamins.

Fat-soluble vitamins are able to be stored in the liver and therefore do not require to be taken in the diet every day. Fat-soluble vitamins are vitamins A, D, E and K.

Water-soluble vitamins cannot be stored by the body and need to be taken regularly as part of the diet. These vitamins include the B vitamin group and vitamin C.

Antioxidants

During the processes of normal metabolism and also in response to chemicals such as pollutants, infections and radiation, highly reactive oxygen radicals are formed. These molecules have free hydrogen atoms, which are extremely reactive with the fatty acids in cell membranes and cause damage to them by causing oxidation to occur. This damage is widely accepted as being the biochemical basis of the origins of cancer and also in the formation of the fatty deposits that cause coronary heart disease.

Antioxidants mop up these free radicals thus preventing these harmful oxidative reactions occurring.

MICRONUTRIENTS

Vitamins	Minerals
Thiamin	Calcium
Riboflavin	Phosphorus
Niacin	Iron
B_6	Magnesium
B_{12}	Sodium
Folate	Potassium
Vitamin C	Chloride
Vitamin A	Zinc
Vitamin D	Copper*
Vitamin E	Selenium*
Vitamin K	Iodine*
	Molybdenum*
	Cobalt*
	Manganese*
	Chromium*
	Fluoride*

* Trace elements

VITAMINS

- **Required in tiny amounts**
  - **Essential for metabolic processes**

- **Fat-soluble**
  - **A (beta-carotene precursor), D, K, E**

- **Water-soluble**

- **C, B group**

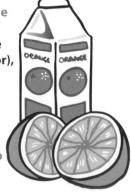

Vitamin C, beta-carotene, vitamin E and the mineral selenium all act as antioxidants and scavenge the free radicals, thus preventing them doing harm. In addition, other antioxidants are found in plants and thus fruit and vegetables; for example, the antioxidant lycopene is found in tomatoes.

WATER-SOLUBLE VITAMINS

B Vitamin group

This group comprises several vitamins. They are called the B Vitamin group and are all water-soluble.

Thiamin (Vitamin B₁)

Vitamin B_1 is called thiamin and is involved in metabolic reactions for energy release from carbohydrates, normal growth in children and the functioning and maintenance of nerves.

Vitamin B_1 is found in red meat, liver, milk, fortified breakfast cereals, potatoes, bread, pasta and yeast extracts. Meat is an important source of B vitamins and pork is a particularly rich source of thiamin.

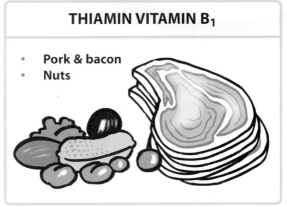

THIAMIN VITAMIN B₁

- **Pork & bacon**
- **Nuts**

The RNI for vitamin B_1 is 0.2 milligrams/day for infants up to 9 months. For infants 10-12 months it is 0.3 milligrams/day, for children 1-3 years it is 0.5 milligrams/day and for children 4-10 years it is 0.7 milligrams/day.

For males aged 11-14 years it is 0.9 milligrams/day, for those 15-18 years it is 1.1 milligrams/day, for those 19-50 years it is 1.0 milligrams/day and for males over 50 years it is 0.9 milligrams/day.

For females aged 11-14 years it is 0.7 milligrams/day, and for those 15 years and over it is 0.8 milligrams/day.

During the last trimester of pregnancy it is 0.1 milligrams/day and during breastfeeding the requirements for vitamin B_1 are increased by 0.2 milligrams/day.

A deficiency called beriberi is seen in developing countries and in the United Kingdom those who suffer from alcoholism may have a deficiency.

Riboflavin (Vitamin B₂)

Vitamin B_2 is called riboflavin. It is a water-soluble vitamin and is involved in metabolic reactions for energy release from foods and for normal growth in children.

Vitamin B_2 is found in red meat, liver, milk and dairy products, fortified breakfast cereals and yeast extracts.

The RNI for vitamin B_2 is 0.4 milligrams/day for infants up to 12 months. For children 1-3 years it is 0.6 milligrams/day, for children 4-6 years it is 0.8 milligrams/day and for children 7-10 years it is 1.0 milligrams/day.

For males aged 11-14 years it is 1.2 milligrams/day, for those 15 and over it is 1.3 milligrams/day.

For females aged 11 years and over it is 1.1 milligrams/day.

During the last trimester of pregnancy the requirements for vitamin B_2 are increased by 0.3 milligrams/day and during breastfeeding the requirement is increased by 0.5 milligrams/day.

A deficiency causing a sore tongue and mouth is seen in third world countries.

Sunlight can destroy B_2 and heating in the presence of bicarbonate of soda (sometimes used in cooking) can also destroy it.

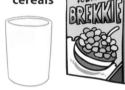

RIBOFLAVIN VITAMIN B_2

- **Dairy produce**
- **Fortified breakfast cereals**

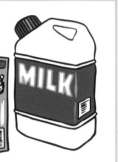

Niacin (Vitamin B_3)

Vitamin B_3 is called niacin or nicotinic acid. It is a water-soluble vitamin and is involved in metabolic reactions for energy release from carbohydrates. Vitamin B_3 is found in red meat, liver, milk and dairy products, fortified breakfast cereals, bread, potatoes, fish and yeast extracts.

The RNI for vitamin B_3 is 3 milligrams/day for infants up to 6 months, and 4 milligrams/day for infants 7-9 months and 5 milligrams/day for infants 10-12 months. For children 1-3 years it is 8 milligrams/day, for children 4-6 years it is 11 milligrams/day and for children 7-10 years it is 12 milligrams/day.

NIACIN VITAMIN B_3

- **Meat & fish**
- **Fortified breakfast cereals**

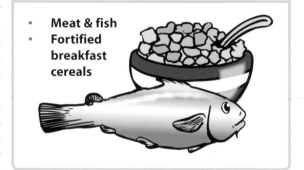

For males aged 11-14 years it is 15 milligrams/day, for those 15-18 years it is 18 milligrams/day, for those 19 -50 years it is 17 milligrams/day and for males over 50 years it is 16 milligrams/day.

For females aged 11-14 years it is 12 milligrams/day, for those 15-18 years it is 14 milligrams/day, for those 19 -50 years it is 13 milligrams/day and for females over 50 years it is 12 milligrams/day.

During pregnancy the requirements for vitamin B_3 are not increased.

During breastfeeding the requirement for vitamin B_3 is increased by 2 milligrams/day.

A deficiency called Pellagra, which causes a rash, is seen in developing countries.

Cooking can affect vitamin B_3 as boiling vegetables cause it to be lost and heat can also destroy it.

Pyridoxine (Vitamin B_6)

Vitamin B_6 is called pyridoxine and is involved in protein metabolism and the formation of red blood cells.

It is found in red meat, liver, fortified breakfast cereals, potatoes, eggs and yeast extracts.

The RNI for vitamin B_1 is 0.2 milligrams/day for infants up to 6 months. For infants 7-9 months it is 0.3 milligrams/day and for those 10-12 months it is 0.4 milligrams/day, for children 1-3 years it is 0.7 milligrams/day, for children 4-6 years it is 0.9 milligrams/day and for children 7-10 years it is 1.0 milligrams/day.

For males aged 11-14 years it is 1.2 milligrams/day, for those 15-18 years it is 1.5 milligrams/day, and for those 19 years and over it is 1.4 milligrams/day.

For females aged 11-14 years it is 1.0 milligrams/day; for those 15 years and over it is 1.2 milligrams/day.

No increase is considered to be needed in pregnancy.

Some people who take large amounts of this vitamin such as some women who take it for the relief of premenstrual tension (PMT) symptoms may experience peripheral nerve problems causing tingling of the fingers and toes. These symptoms are reversible and cease when the supplements are discontinued.

PYRIDOXINE VITAMIN B$_6$

- Meat & fish
- Eggs
- Whole grains
- Fortified breakfast cereals

Cobalamin or Cyanocobalamin (Vitamin B$_{12}$)

Vitamin B$_{12}$ or cobalamin is required for the formation of red blood cells and without adequate quantities of it in the diet a type of anaemia can result due to the formation of incorrect red blood cells.

Red meat is a major source of vitamin B$_{12}$ or cobalamin. This vitamin is only found in foods of animal origin such as milk, meat and eggs. It is also found in yeast.

Therefore if no meat or eggs are taken in the diet, it is important to include a source of vitamin B$_{12}$ such as that from dairy products. Those who do not take red meat such as vegetarians and those who take no products of animal origin such as vegans need to ensure they take enough of this important vitamin from another source such as yeasts or as a supplement.

COBALAMIN VITAMIN B$_{12}$

- Offal & meat
- Dairy produce

Folate

Folate is one of the range of B vitamins and like all B vitamins is water-soluble. Folate is important for the formation of blood cells and also is particularly recommended during early pregnancy to prevent neural tube defects such as spina bifida. Any woman who is considering becoming pregnant is encouraged to take plenty of folate-rich foods in her diet. Women who are pregnant are prescribed a supplement of folic acid for the first few weeks of pregnancy.

Folate is mainly found in leafy green vegetables such as sprouts, spinach, green beans and peas. Potatoes and fruit such as oranges also contain folate.

Ascorbic acid (Vitamin C)

Ascorbic acid or vitamin C is water-soluble and is found in all types of fruit and vegetables. It is required for healing to occur and necessary for the integrity of connective tissue. It is also an important antioxidant vitamin and as such it helps the body to resist diseases and infections by maximising the functioning of the immune system.

Especially rich sources of vitamin C are citrus fruits such as oranges and grapefruit as well as berry fruits like blackberries. Vegetables are also good sources especially green vegetables, peppers and tomatoes. Even potatoes contain vitamin C. Thus potatoes can make a substantial contribution to vitamin C in the diet.

To maximise the amount of vitamin C in vegetables they should be cooked in a minimum amount of water and kept warm for a minimum amount of time. A deficiency of vitamin C causes scurvy.

> ### ASCORBIC ACID VITAMIN C
>
> - **Citrus & soft fruits**
> - **Fruit juice**
> - **Potatoes, green vegetables & salad**

FAT-SOLUBLE VITAMINS

Retinol (Vitamin A)

Vitamin A or retinol is a fat-soluble vitamin. It can be formed in the body from its precursor beta-carotene. (A precursor is a substance that the body needs to convert into another substance.)

Vitamin A is required for vision, and is involved in making a pigment which is formed in the retina of the eye and enables one to see in dim light. It is also needed for the maintenance of a healthy skin and mucous membranes and normal growth in children.

> ### RETINOL VITAMIN A
>
> - **Liver**
> - **Oily fish (e.g. herrings) & cod liver oil**
> - **Dairy produce**
> - **Beta-carotene – precursor**
> - **Carrots & green leafy vegetables**
> - **Peaches, nectarines & dried apricots**

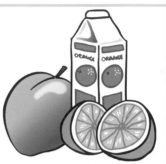

Vitamin A is found in full fat milk, cheese, eggs, oily fish, liver and butter. Vitamin A is added to margarines and spreads.

It is also formed from beta-carotene, which is found in carrots, spinach, apricots, tomatoes and cabbage. Carotenes give the yellowish-orange colour found in fruit and vegetables.

Carotene is an oxidant and, like vitamin C, has a positive effect on enhancing the immune system.

The RNI for Vitamin A is 350 micrograms/day for infants up to 12 months. For children 1-3 years it is 400 micrograms/day, for children 4-10 years it is 500 micrograms/day.

For males aged 11-14 years it is 600 micrograms/day, 15 years and over, it is 700 micrograms/day.

For females aged 11 and over, it is 600 micrograms/day.

During pregnancy the requirement increases by 100 micrograms/day. It should be remembered that an excess of vitamin A during pregnancy is thought to be harmful to the growing foetus. For that reason liver and vitamin A supplements are not recommended during pregnancy. During breastfeeding the requirements for vitamin A are increased by 350 micrograms/day.

Too much vitamin A can be harmful, because, as it is fat-soluble, an excess of it can be stored in the liver. People who cannot digest and absorb fat may need to have vitamin A administered by injection. Deficiencies of vitamin A are common in developing countries and may cause growth retardation in children and blindness.

Cholecalciferol (Vitamin D)

Vitamin D is fat-soluble and is required by the body to enable calcium absorption to occur in the small intestine. Thus bone health is related to adequate calcium and vitamin D during the growing years.

Most people derive vitamin D by the action of sunlight on the skin. Vitamin D is also derived from meat and fish, butter, full cream milk and eggs. It is added to low fat spreads and margarines. Lean red meat has been shown to be a valuable source of vitamin D.

For those who wear clothing that covers the body and who do not take meat or fish an alternative source of vitamin D is needed. Without adequate vitamin D in the diet, calcium cannot be properly absorbed and the bones become weak which results in the condition of rickets in children and osteomalacia in adults. Toddlers suffering from rickets have bone pain and bowed legs, while teenagers suffer from bone pain and knock knees.

> ## CHOLECALCIFEROL VITAMIN D
>
> - **Sunlight**
>
> **Food sources are few but include:**
> - **Oily fish & cod liver oil**
> - **Eggs, meat**
> - **Margarine**
> - **Fortified breakfast cereals**

Tocopherol (Vitamin E)

Vitamin E or tocopherol is a fat-soluble vitamin. It is widely available in foods and acts as an anti-oxidant. Antioxidants help to protect the body from diseases. Vitamin E is needed for healthy membranes. There is also increasing evidence that vitamin E may protect against heart disease and cancer.

Vitamin E is widely available and is often found in polyunsaturated oils such as soya oil. Therefore it is found in vegetable oils, margarines, oily fish such as sardines, wholegrains, cereals, green leafy vegetables, nuts and seeds.

There is no RNI for Vitamin E.

> ## TOCOPHEROL VITAMIN E
>
> - **Vegetable oils**
> - **Nuts**
> - **Eggs**
> - **Whole-grain cereals**
> - **Avocados & leafy green vegetables**

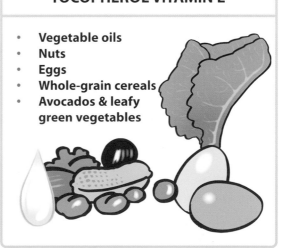

VITAMIN K

- **Whole-grain cereals**
- **Leafy green vegetables**

Vitamin K

Vitamin K is a fat-soluble vitamin. It can be formed in the body by bacterial synthesis in the intestinal tract. It is required for the correct clotting of blood. There are billions of bacteria in the digestive tract and these can help to produce vitamin K.

Vitamin K is found in leafy green vegetables such as spinach and cabbage. Red meat, cereals and oils also contain vitamin K.

There is no RNI for Vitamin K as it is widely distributed in foods. ·

Deficiencies are rarely seen but occasionally newborn babies have a deficiency.

MINERALS

The minerals calcium, phosphorus, iron, magnesium, sodium, potassium, chlorine, and zinc are all essential minerals. The minerals copper, selenium, iodine, molybdenum and cobalt are all also essential but as they are needed in tiny amounts they are called trace minerals or elements.

Calcium

Calcium combines with phosphorus to make calcium phosphate, which is the chief material that gives hardness and strength to bones and teeth. It is required for part of the complex mechanism which causes blood to clot after an injury. It is also required for the correct functioning of muscles and nerves and also for the maintenance of bones and teeth once formed.

Calcium is found in good supply in milk, cheese, bread (added to white flour by law), bones of canned fish and hard water.

CALCIUM

- **Cheese, yoghurt & milk**
- **Dark green leafy vegetables**
- **White bread & fortified flour**
- **Canned fish (if bones are eaten)**

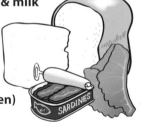

The absorption of calcium (and phosphorous) and the mineralisation (deposition of the calcium and phosphorus) of bones and teeth is controlled by vitamin D.

Calcium deficiency in children means that bones and teeth are not mineralised properly and are improperly formed. The leg bones may bend under the weight of the body as in rickets. In adults the strength in bones and teeth is not maintained possibly resulting in osteomalacia (adult rickets). Muscles and nerves do not function correctly which may result in a condition called tetany.

Phosphorus

Phosphorus works in conjunction with calcium and therefore has the same functions and also gives structure to bones and teeth.

In addition it is important because it is a vital component for the production of energy in the body.

Phosphorus is present as phosphate in all plant and animal cells and is therefore present in all natural foods. It forms part of many proteins and is often used as an additive in manufactured foods. Additives such as phosphates are used as emulsifiers and stabilisers in foodstuffs.

A normal diet will supply sufficient phosphorus for all age groups. The requirement of phosphorus is linked with that of calcium in molecular quantities

The RNI for phosphorus is 400 milligrams/day for infants up to 12 months. For children 1-3 years it is 270 milligrams/day, children 4-6 years it is 350 milligrams/day, and children 7-10 years it is 450 milligrams/day.

For males aged 11-18 years it is 775 milligrams/day; 19 years plus it is 550 milligrams/day.

For females aged 11-18 years it is 625 milligrams/day, and for those of 19 years and over it is 550 milligrams/day.

During breastfeeding the requirements for phosphorus are increased by 440 milligrams/day.

Some people with kidney problems (renal disease) may need to limit the amount of phosphorus they take. A deficiency of phosphorus is not known to occur.

Iron

Iron is an essential nutrient. It acts as an oxygen carrier in the blood and muscle. A lack of dietary iron can contribute to iron deficiency anaemia.

Iron deficiency anaemia is one of the most common nutritional deficiencies

IRON
• **Offal & red meat**
• **Dark green vegetables**
• **Pulses & whole-grain cereals**
• **Nuts & seeds**
• **Fortified breakfast cereals**
• **Ground spices & dried herbs**

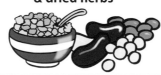
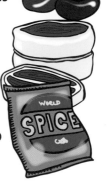

SOURCES OF IRON

Haem-iron is easily absorbed

Found in:
• **Red meat (beef, pork and lamb)**
• **Offal (liver and kidney)**
• **Fish**

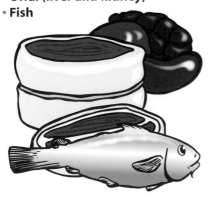

and particularly affects infants between 6 and 12 months, teenagers especially girls, women of menstruating age and elderly people.

There are two forms of dietary iron: haem-iron and non-haem iron. The iron in red meat is in the haem form, and is well absorbed while the iron in cereals, vegetables and fruit is poorly absorbed. However, if meat is eaten at the same meal as other foods then it actually enhances the absorption of iron from these other foods. Vitamin C helps the absorption of iron in the non-haem form.

For iron the RNI for adult men aged 19-50 years is 8.7 milligrams/day and for adult women of the same age it is 14.8 milligrams/day. A 100g portion of cooked beef braising steak would provide 31% of the adult man's requirement for iron and 18% of the adult woman's requirement for iron. Thus red meat provides a valuable contribution to the amount of iron in the diet.

Magnesium

Magnesium is needed for the development of the skeleton and for the functioning of nerves.

It is present in chlorophyll, the green colouring matter in plants. Therefore vegetables are a source of magnesium. Red meat also contains magnesium. Epsom salts are based on magnesium.

SOURCES OF IRON

Non-haem iron less easily absorbed

Found in:
• **Pulses (peas, dried beans and lentils)**
• **Eggs**
• **Nuts**
• **Dried fruit**
• **Chocolate**

MAGNESIUM

• **Whole grain**
• **Nuts & cereals**
• **Green vegetables**
• **Tap water (in hard water areas)**

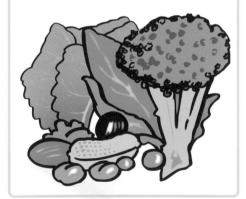

The RNI for magnesium is 55 milligrams/day for infants up to 3 months. For infants 4-6 months it is 60 milligrams/day, for infants 7-9 months it is 75 milligrams/day and for infants 10-12 months it is 80 milligrams/day. For children 1-3 years it is 85 milligrams/day, for children 4-6 years it is 120 milligrams/day and for children 7-10 years it is 200 milligrams/day.

For males and females aged 11-14 years it is 280 milligrams/day. For males and females aged 15-18 years it is 300 milligrams/day.

For males 19 years and over it is 300 milligrams/day.

For females 19 years and over it is 270 milligrams/day.

During lactation an extra 50 milligrams/day is required.

Sodium

Sodium is called an electrolyte as together with potassium and chloride it helps to maintain the fluid balance in the body. Sodium is also required for nerve and muscle impulses. Most sodium is found in the fluid outside the cells.

Sodium is easily absorbed by the body and excess sodium in the diet is linked to high blood pressure. The kidneys control the level of sodium in the blood by excreting excess in the urine. Due to the immaturity of babies' kidneys they cannot tolerate a high level of sodium in the diet. Sodium is also lost in the sweat and therefore in those working in a hot climate or undertaking very strenuous activity an excessive loss of sweat can lead to muscle cramps.

Sodium is a major component of table salt (sodium chloride). There is approximately 1 gram of sodium in each 2.5 grams of sodium chloride. Sodium chloride is used extensively in cooking to bring out the flavour of foods and also added to food at the table. Snacks such as crisps and savoury biscuits are popular and contribute to the sodium intake. Canned foods also contains increased levels of salt compared with fresh or frozen foods.

Traditionally salt has been used as a preservative for pickles and in salting fish and meat.

Sodium is a component of many additives, used in the manufacture of processed foods. Examples of these are Monosodium Glutamate (MSG), a flavour enhancer used in soups and ready prepared meals. MSG is also traditionally used in Chinese cooking.

Sodium nitrite is used as a preservative in producing bacon, and ham also contains sodium.

As can be seen, processed foods have higher levels of sodium in them than fresh foods such as fresh fruit and vegetables, fresh meat and fish and cereals such as rice.

The RNI for sodium for adults is 1,600 milligrams (1.6g) per day. Yet the average intake from the diet is 3.5g of sodium per day, which is more than twice the RNI. This 3.5g of sodium per day equates with about 9 g per day of salt. It is recommended that as a population we should cut our salt consumption by a third. This means that we should aim for a maximum intake of 6g of salt per day.

Excessive sodium consumption is associated with high blood pressure. Afro-Caribbean people and also those with diabetes are particularly prone to high blood pressure or hypertension as it is correctly called. Factors such as obesity also contribute to raised blood pressure.

Hypertension increases the incidence of strokes and heart disease and therefore a reduction in sodium intake by the population generally is considered to have a beneficial effect in reducing these health problems.

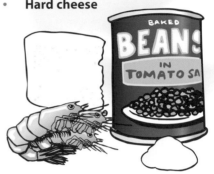

SODIUM

- **Salt**
- **Prawns**
- **Baked beans in tomato sauce**
- **Hard cheese**

Potassium

Like sodium, potassium is an electrolyte and is involved in the fluid balance of the body. It is found inside the cells in intracellular fluid.

Potassium can counter the effects of sodium to an extent in helping to lower blood pressure. Therefore a diet high in potassium is advocated for the majority of the population.

Potassium is required for the correct functioning of the muscles of the heart. In severe cases of depletion of potassium, heart failure may result.

As with sodium, the majority of potassium in the diet is absorbed and any excess excreted by the kidneys. Some people who have to take medicines such as diuretics may excrete too much potassium and may thus require potassium supplements to balance the effects. People with severe diarrhoea may also lose excessive amounts of potassium.

The main dietary sources of potassium are fruit and vegetables but potassium is particularly prevalent in bananas, fruit juices, coffee and potatoes. Low salt substitutes are based on potassium rather than sodium.

POTASSIUM

- Bananas
- All other fruits & vegetables

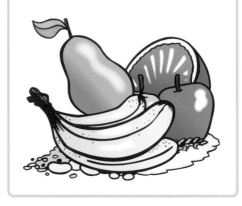

Chloride

Chloride is found along with sodium in the extracellular fluid and all other body fluids such as blood. Like sodium and potassium it is an electrolyte.

Most chloride is assimilated into the body along with sodium in sodium chloride (table salt).

Chloride is also part of the hydrochloric acid produced by the stomach and needed for digestion there.

Zinc

Zinc is a vital component in the functioning of the immune system of the body, which helps to fight diseases and infections. Zinc is also needed for the healing of wounds. It is also involved in the development of sexual maturity, particularly in males.

The most reliable source of zinc in the diet is from meat which is in a form which is easily absorbed.

For zinc the RNI for adult men aged 19-50 years is 9.5 milligrams/day and for adult women of the same age it is 7.0 milligrams/day.

A 100g portion of cooked pork leg joint, roasted medium, lean contains 3.2 milligrams/day zinc. Therefore this provides 34% of the adult man's requirement for zinc and 46% of the adult woman's requirement for zinc.

ZINC

- Meat
- Dairy products
- Pulses & whole grain cereals

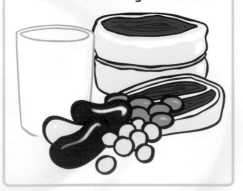

Copper

Copper is a component of many of the enzyme systems in the body.

It is found in liver, shellfish, meat, bread, cereals and vegetables. Some people with rheumatoid arthritis wear copper bracelets to help relieve their symptoms as some copper is absorbed through the skin. Babies who are fed for too long a period on cows' milk may occasionally show a deficiency of copper.

The RNI for copper is 0.2 milligrams/day for infants up to 3 months. For infants 4 months to 12 months it is 0.3 milligrams/day, for children 1-3 years it is 0.4 milligrams/day, for children 4-6 years it is 0.6 milligrams/day and for children 7-10 years it is 0.7 milligrams/day.

For males and females aged 11-14 years it is 0.8 milligrams/day, for those aged 15-18 years it is 1.0 milligrams/day, for those aged 19 years and over it is 1.2 milligrams/day.

During lactation an extra 0.3 milligrams/day is needed.

COPPER

- **Nuts**
- **Cereals**
- **Potatoes & other vegetables**
- **Meat**

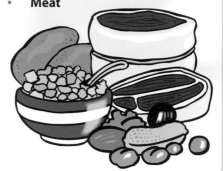

Selenium

Selenium is an important antioxidant and, like other antioxidants, has a protective effect against heart disease.

Selenium is found naturally in red meat. Fish and cereals contain selenium. Red meat is a good source of selenium. It is considered to be important in protecting against coronary heart disease and cancers.

In areas where the soil is low in selenium then cereals can have a reduced content of selenium. Brazil nuts are a rich source of selenium.

Excessive amounts of selenium can be taken by taking too many supplements containing it.

The RNI for selenium is 10 micrograms/day for infants up to 3 months. For infants 4-6 months it is 13 micrograms/day and from 7 to 12 months it is 10 micrograms/day; for children 1-3 years it is 15 micrograms/day.

SELENIUM

- **Brazil nuts**
- **Fish**
- **Seeds**
- **Offal**

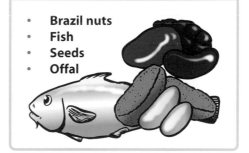

For children 4-6 years it is 20 micrograms/day and children 7-10 years it is 30 micrograms/day.

For males and females aged 11-14 years the RNI is 45 micrograms/day.

For males aged 15-18 years it is 70 micrograms/day. For males over 19 years it is 75 micrograms/day.

For females over 15 years it is 60 micrograms/day. During lactation an extra 15 micrograms/day is required.

Fluoride

Fluoride has been shown to be an important factor in the strengthening of teeth against decay. It is thought that it combines with the protective enamel coating of the teeth thus making them more resistant to attack by the acid produced by bacteria in the mouth. For this reason fluoride has been added to drinking water and toothpastes.

Fluoride is found naturally in tea, sea water fish and, in some parts of the country, in water supplies. Tea provides most of the fluoride in the diet in this country.

In areas of the country where fluoride occurs naturally in the water supply the number of children who require treatment for tooth decay is known to be significantly lower than in other areas. Because of this it has been recommended that all water supplies should have fluoride added to them.

One part per million of fluoride is added to water to assist in preventing dental decay.

Excessive amounts of fluoride can cause mottling of the teeth. Excessive amounts of fluoride can be taken by taking too many supplements containing fluoride. There is no RNI for fluoride.

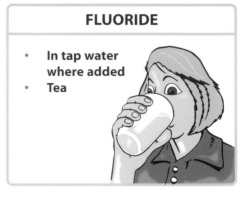

FLUORIDE

- **In tap water where added**
- **Tea**

Iodine

Iodine is required to make the hormone thyroxine which is produced by the thyroid gland in the neck. Thyroxine along with other hormones helps to control the rate of metabolism in the body.

Iodine is widely distributed in foods but is found in good supply in seafoods, milk, green vegetables – especially spinach, fresh water (depending upon area) and iodised salt (added commercially).

A deficiency of iodine leads to a reduction in

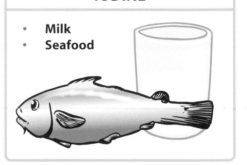

IODINE

- **Milk**
- **Seafood**

the amount of thyroxine produced by the thyroid gland. As a result the metabolism slows down and the gland swells up. This swelling can be seen in the neck and is called a goitre. Such swellings were commonly found in people in Switzerland and Derbyshire in the past.

The RNI for iodine is 50 micrograms/day for infants up to 3 months. For infants 4-12 months it is 60 micrograms/day, for children 1-3 years it is 70 micrograms/day, for children 4-6 years it is 100 micrograms/day and for those 7-10 years it is 110 micrograms/day.

For males and females aged 11-14 years it is 130 micrograms/day, for those 15 years plus it is 140 micrograms/day.

Manganese

This is a trace element needed for certain enzymes. It is found widely in foods.

Chromium

This is a trace element needed in glucose metabolism. It is found in a variety of foods.

Molybdenum

This is required for the activation of certain enzymes in the body and is widely found in foods.

Cobalt

Cobalt in found in vitamin B_{12}, which is needed for red blood cell formation.

WHERE MICRONUTRIENTS ARE FOUND IN THE DIET OF PEOPLE IN THE UK

Food sources of the micronutrients that may be present in sufficient amounts in the diets of some people.

	MAIN SOURCES OF NUTRIENTS
VITAMIN A	Vegetables (excluding potatoes); milk and milk products; meat and meat products half of which came from liver; fat spreads; cereal and cereal products.
RIBOFLAVIN	Milk and milk products; cereal and cereal products; meat and meat products.
FOLATE	Cereal and cereal products; vegetables, potatoes and savoury snacks; milk and milk products.
ZINC	Meat and meat products; cereal and cereal products; milk and milk products; vegetables, potatoes and savoury snacks.
IRON	Cereal and cereal products, particularly breakfast cereals and bread; vegetables, potatoes and savoury snacks; meat and meat products.
MAGNESIUM	Cereal and cereal products; vegetables, potatoes and savoury snacks, over half of which came from potatoes; milk and milk products; meat and meat products.
CALCIUM	Milk and milk products; cereal and cereal products, particularly bread.
POTASSIUM	Vegetables, potatoes and savoury snacks, with two thirds coming from potatoes; milk and milk products; cereal and cereal products; meat and meat products.
IODINE	Milk and milk products; cereal and cereal products; fish and fish dishes.

Question to determine progress

Write notes on Vitamin C and Iron. **See answer in the appendix.**

5 Fluids including alcohol

Why we need fluid

Fluid is absolutely vital to life. Without adequate fluid we would only live a few days; without food but with an adequate supply of water, survival can be for several months.

About fifty to seventy percent of the body is fluid, or body water, and all of the vital actions that occur in the body take place in a liquid environment. The electrolytes sodium and potassium help to control fluid balance in the body. Fluid is needed in the body for:

1. Various solvent molecules in the body such as digestive enzymes.
2. Transport medium such as blood.
3. Lubricant such as the synovial fluid in joints.
4. Regulation of body temperature.

The percentage of body water is greater in infants than adults. Also because women have greater stores of body fat than men they have proportionally less body water.

The digestive process requires copious amounts of digestive fluids to be produced. Fluid is absorbed throughout the digestive tract but the majority of fluid is re-absorbed in the colon.

Body water

Body water comprises intracellular (fluid inside the cells) and extracellular components (fluid outside the cell).

Fluid passes between the two areas via the semi-permeable cell membrane. Potassium is found within the cell and sodium outside of it.

Fluid is taken in drinks and also in foodstuffs. Some foods have a greater proportion of fluid than others. For example, fruit and vegetables as well as soups and jellies have a high percentage of water in them. Small quantities of water are also produced during the metabolic reactions that occur in the body.

The kidneys are the major organ responsible for excreting fluid and also waste products of metabolism in the urine. Fluid is also lost from the body in the faeces, exhaled air and in sweat.

Obviously in hot climates more sweat is produced and the evaporation of this from the skin helps to regulate the body temperature.

The regulation of fluid balance is under tight control. If the extracellular fluid becomes more concentrated then hormones are secreted by the hypothalamus in the brain and this stimulates the sensation of thirst as well as greater re-absorption of fluid in the kidneys.

All adults and teenagers need approximately 2 litres (about 3 pints) of fluid per day to meet their requirements. Yet it is not unusual to find that people take too little fluid.

Problems with a lack of fluid

Lack of fluid can result in numerous problems, including tiredness and irritability.

A lack of concentration in lessons and poor attention spans can be attributed to lack of fluid. Dry skin can also be due to lack of fluid.

Medical problems such as urinary tract infections and disorders of the gastro-intestinal tract such as irritable bowel syndrome can all be partly due to inadequate fluid intake.

Hot weather or being in warm environments such as car or coach journeys or in warm classrooms or laboratories, can all increase fluid losses from the body as perspiration increases.

Games, dancing or any other extra activity result in extra losses of fluid. These increased losses all need to be replenished by drinking more fluid.

Thirst is the body's way of telling us to drink. If we feel thirsty it means that we are already suffering about 2% dehydration. Often thirst is ignored and dehydration increases.

Sport

For those who take part in active sports, fluid can make the difference between winning and losing the race or a match. Nowadays at any sports event, fluid is taken before and afterwards. Again, not only does adequate fluid help with the physical performance but it also helps with concentration and alertness, which can result in winning or being a runner-up.

The National Nutritional Standards for School Lunches

The National Nutritional Standards for School Lunches, which were published in 2000 by the Department for Education and Employment, do not have any compulsory standards as regards fluid.

They do have an additional recommendation that the Secretary of State:

♦   expects drinking water should be available to all children every day free of charge; and
♦   strongly recommends that drinking milk is available as an option every day.

In the section on planning the menu it recommends that unsweetened fruit juice be offered as a drink option.

Water

The obvious fluid to take to replace fluid is water. This can be either as tap water or bottled water. Water can be taken straight from the tap or filtered and chilled. Filtering removes substances such as nitrates, which may be present.

If bottled water is used this can be either the still or carbonated varieties. If large bottles of water are used, it is important that they are drunk within a day because bottled water does not usually contain chlorine which helps to protect tap water from bacteria.

Flavoured waters are popular but some contain large amounts of sugar.

Milk

Milk and drinks based on milk, such as milk shakes, are an important source of calcium, which is needed for the development of strong and healthy bones. Indeed it is during the teenage years that most of the calcium is deposited in the bones. Thus this is a very important time for developing a strong skeleton. Milk is also a good source of protein needed for the synthesis of tissues such as muscles, vital organs, skin, blood and digestive enzymes.

Skimmed milk is not suitable for children under five years of age as it does not contain enough calories. Full cream milk should be used for children up to two years of age when semi-skimmed milk can be introduced.

Children can be tempted to drink more milk by clever marketing, such as is seen with the 'White stuff' promotion. Providing cold milk with cereals at breakfast clubs and at mid-morning break is popular.

Yoghurt drinks also contain calcium and can be popular with young people. Fruit 'smoothies' containing puréed fruits and yoghurt have increased in popularity.

Some children and adults are allergic or intolerant to cows' milk. This intolerance usually begins soon after birth. Most children grow out of this intolerance to cows' milk by the age of five years. Unfortunately for some this intolerance persists throughout life. Such children must not be given cows' milk. Soya milk or specially prescribed milks should be provided instead. Any soya milk used should be one of the brands supplemented with extra calcium.

Fruit juices and squashes

Fruit juices contain vitamin C, which is important to health as it acts as an antioxidant. Juices are popular especially with young people and indeed can provide substantial amounts of vitamin C. It is recommended that juices without added sugar are provided.

Low sugar squashes can be useful in providing fluid in an acceptable form to youngsters and adults alike. Most squashes now do not contain additives or colours, which were implicated in hyperactivity in some children.

Tea, coffees, malted milk and hot chocolate

Tea and coffees are popular hot drinks and they provide a way of including milk. Cappuccinos can be popular and a useful way of encouraging milk consumption. Unfortunately it has been found that teenage girls often do not take enough calcium and any drinks that encourage them to take more calcium can only be beneficial.

Both ordinary tea and coffees contain caffeine, but decaffeinated varieties can be provided. It has been found that tea contains antioxidants, which are considered to help to prevent heart disease. Herb teas are also increasingly popular and contain no caffeine. Hot chocolate is very popular in cold weather, and the low sugar varieties can be provided.

Malted milks can be popular with children and elderly people at bedtime and are a way of providing extra milk.

Colas, lemonades and other fizzy drinks

These are often popular with children but can be a source of sugar. Indeed a survey showed that they were the most common drinks consumed by young people. The majority of the young people taking them chose the sugar-containing variety. Constantly drinking these can have a detrimental effect on dental health due to the sugar they contain.

Colas are especially popular and like tea and coffee contain caffeine. They can also provide a lot of sugar, and sugar-free varieties may be a preferable option. If sugary colas are chosen in preference to sugar free varieties, they are best consumed at mealtimes to limit the effect on dental health.

Slush drinks

Highly coloured slush drinks have gained popularity with children. They can be a way of providing fluid but can be rich in sugar and additives especially food colours.

Soups and hot drinks

'Cup-a-soups' and savoury drinks can be popular during cold weather. Obviously they can be a source of salt.

Home-made soups are unlikely to contain as much salt.

Caffeine

This is found in teas, coffees, colas and chocolate. Caffeine acts as a diuretic and causes the kidney to excrete more fluid. Caffeine can also have an effect on behaviour causing people to be more alert, but an excess can make them tense.

Alcohol

Alcohol is quickly absorbed from the stomach and from the small intestine. Due to this rapid absorption the effects of intoxication may be quickly experienced.

Alcohol is a rich source of calories and each gram of alcohol provides 7 kcals. Therefore alcohol consumption can contribute to obesity and this is seen in many middle-aged men who have excessive fat deposition around their stomachs due to over-consumption of beer.

Like caffeine, alcohol has a diuretic effect.

ALCOHOL

- **Beer/lager/cider**   3-6% alcohol
- **Wines**   9-13% alcohol
- **Spirits**   37-45% alcohol
- **Liqueurs**   20-40% alcohol
- **Fortified wines**   18-25% alcohol

- **Absorbed in stomach**

- **Broken down in liver**

- **7 calories per gram**

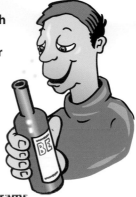

- **Unit of alcohol = 8 grams**

  - **Half pint of beer/lager/cider (300ml)**
  - **Glass of wine (100ml)**
  - **Tot of spirits (25ml)**

Units of alcohol

In order to encourage people to limit their alcohol consumption to a sensible level, the concept of units of alcohol has been produced.

A unit of alcohol is basically the amount of an alcoholic beverage that contains a given amount of alcohol. The following contain a unit of alcohol:

- small pub-size glass of wine;
- half pint beer;
- half pint larger;
- half pint cider;
- schooner of sherry; and
- tot of spirits such as brandy, whisky, gin, rum or vodka.

It is recommended that adults limit their alcohol intake to sensible levels. Women are recommended not to take more than 2 or 3 units of alcohol per day and men 3-4 units of alcohol per day. It is recommended that the alcoholic drinks are not saved up and drunk in one binge session. Also it is recommended that everyone has at least one alcohol-free day each week.

Alcoholism and effects on the liver

Alcohol can be addictive and many people have become alcoholics with the accompanying health problems of liver cirrhosis.

Alcohol is detoxified and broken down by the liver. It does this at the rate of one unit of alcohol per hour. Because women have a smaller liver than men their tolerance for alcohol is less.

Excessive quantities of alcohol taken regularly impose an enormous burden on the liver and eventually the cells of the liver fail to be able to cope with alcohol and become replaced by fat and scar tissues. This occurs in liver cirrhosis.

Question to determine progress

What are the maximum recommended amounts of alcohol that should be taken per week? Briefly mention the health risks associated with excessive alcohol consumption. **See answer in the appendix.**

6 The fate of nutrients

When food is eaten, the nutrients it contains are used for a number of processes in the body:
1.   Carbohydrate is used for energy.
2.   Dietary fibre or NSP is used for providing bulk to the diet and assisting the passage of the waste products of digestion to be eliminated from the body.
3.   Protein is used for replacement, repair and growth of body tissues. It can also be used for energy.
4.   Fat is used for energy. Also essential fatty acids are used for the formation of cell membranes and hormones.
5.   Alcohol is used for energy, but it can also act as a toxin (poison) to liver cells.
6.   Minerals are used to replace and repair body tissues and regulate body processes.
7.   Vitamins regulate body processes.
8.   Fluid is required as an major component of all body cells for fluid systems such as the blood, lymph and digestive fluids.

No matter what type of food is eaten, the nutrients it contains cannot be used by the body for any of these functions until they enter the bloodstream of the body.

DIGESTION

This is the process whereby food is broken down into its component nutrients.   For example:

♦   protein is broken down firstly to polypeptides (chains of amino acids), peptides (short chains of amino acids) and then finally amino acids;
♦   carbohydrates are broken down into monosaccharides before absorption; and
♦   fats are broken down to fatty acids.

Digestion occurs in the digestive tract which is some times referred to as the gut or gastrointestinal tract.

For this breakdown of foods into the component nutrients, digestive enzymes are required to work on the bonds between the nutrient molecules.

Before the digestive enzymes work, the foods need to be broken down into smaller pieces and also well mixed with the digestive enzymes produced.

Digestive enzymes are themselves proteins and are secreted by different parts of the digestive tract.

DIGESTIVE TRACT

Digestive tract and small intestine

FOOD

Villi

Blood Vessels

Under a microscope the small intestine looks like this.

Food is absorbed into the blood system through the villi.

Mouth

Oesophagus

Liver

Stomach

Gall bladder

Pancreas

Large intestine

Small intestine

Anus

Absorption

Once the foods are broken down into the basic components by the process of digestion these tiny molecules, for example, amino acids, can pass into the blood stream.

This process occurs in the villi of the small intestine. The villi are tiny finger-like projections which thus give the small intestine a vast surface area. Inside each of the villi are blood capillaries.

Nutrients are absorbed across the surface of the villi into the capillaries and hence into the bloodstream.

Digestive tract

The digestive tract consists of various parts:

♦ the mouth, where food is chewed;
♦ the oesophagus, the tube via which the food enters the stomach;
♦ the liver, which secretes bile salts and breaks down toxins such as alcohol;
♦ the gall bladder, which acts as a reservoir for bile salts;
♦ the stomach, which acts as a reservoir for food;
♦ the pancreas, which secretes digestive enzymes;
♦ the small intestine, which consists of the duodenum, jejunum and ileum;
♦ the large intestine or colon; and
♦ the anus, via which the waste products are evacuated.

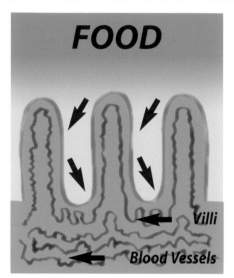

VILLI

FOOD

Villi

Blood Vessels

Under a microscope the small intestine looks like this.

Food is absorbed into the blood system through the villi.

PROCESS OF DIGESTION

Mouth

Here the teeth bite and grind the food into small pieces by the action of chewing. These pieces are small enough to swallow. This breakdown in size of foodstuffs is called 'physical breakdown of food'.

The salivary glands produce saliva to moisten food and make it easy to swallow. The presence of food in the mouth causes the salivary glands to produce saliva. Also the anticipation of food and the sight and smell of it can cause the 'mouth to water' as saliva is produced.

Salivary amylase is produced by the salivary glands and converts some of the cooked starch in food to maltose.

Oesophagus

Food is transported down this tube to the stomach. No digestion occurs in the oesophagus.

Stomach

Food enters the stomach from the oesophagus via a cardiac sphincter. This sphincter is a ring of muscles which protects the entrance to the stomach.

The stomach holds food for 3-4 hours and strong muscular waves and contractions of the stomach move the food and break it down into a soup-like substance called chyme. The food is also mixed with gastric juices produced by the wall of the stomach.

These gastric juices include:

- weak hydrochloric acid produced by the stomach walls, which stops the action of salivary amylase. The hydrochloric acid also helps to destroy some food-poisoning bacteria. About three litres of dilute hydrochloric acid are produced each day;
- the digestive enzyme pepsin, produced by the stomach walls, which starts the breakdown of proteins into peptides and then amino acids;
- rennin, produced in the stomach of young animals and human babies. This enzyme clots milk protein; and
- a substance called intrinsic factor, which is needed for the absorption of vitamin B_{12}.

Food is released from the stomach into the small intestine via the pyloric sphincter.

Small intestine

No further physical breakdown of food occurs in the small intestine. The small intestine is about three metres in length and consists of the duodenum, jejunum and ileum.

In the small intestine most of the digestion and absorption of food occurs.

In the duodenum, bile produced by the liver and which has been stored in the gall bladder is shed onto food. Bile salts emulsify fats into small droplets of fat, which can then be digested.

Pancreatic juices are also poured on to food in the duodenum. Pancreatic juice contains a number of digestive enzymes:

- lipase, which splits fats into fatty acids;
- trypsin, which splits proteins into peptides and amino-acids;
- chymotrypsin, which also splits proteins into peptides and amino acids; and
- amylase, which splits starch into maltose.

The walls of the small intestine also secrete digestive enzymes. These are:

- maltase, which breaks maltose into the component glucose units;
- sucrase, which breaks sucrose into glucose and fructose; and
- lactase, which splits lactose into galactose and glucose.

Some people may not be able to secrete certain digestive enzymes such as lactase, which means they are then unable to tolerate lactose (the sugar found in milk). People from the Middle East are particularly prone to lactase intolerance.

Large intestine or colon

This is the area of the digestive tract where most of the water from foods and beverages is absorbed.

Substances such as dietary fibre or non-starch-polysaccharide (NSP) are resistant to digestion as the digestive enzymes are unable to break the bonds found in fibres. This fibre then gives bulk to the waste products of digestion called faeces and allows them to be easily evacuated from the body via the anus.

Bacteria in the large intestine are able to synthesise vitamin K and some B vitamins.

Absorption

Mouth

No real absorption occurs here due to the short time that food remains in the mouth.

Oesophagus

No absorption occurs.

Stomach

Some absorption of water and alcohol occurs. The absorption of water-soluble vitamins i.e. B vitamins and vitamin C, also occurs.

Small intestine

In the small intestine most absorption of food occurs.

Glucose, other monosaccharides, some dipeptides (units of two amino acids linked together), amino acids, water-soluble vitamins and minerals are absorbed into the blood in the capillaries of the villi.

Vitamin B_{12} is absorbed in the small intestine and intrinsic factor is needed for this process of absorption to occur.

Fatty acids pass through the villi intestinal wall and are rebuilt there into triglycerides which are carried in the lymphatic fluids to the blood supply and then to the liver. Fat-soluble vitamins are absorbed along with the fatty acids.

Large intestine or colon

Here most fluid is absorbed.

The passage of food from mouth to anus is called the transit time and can be 1-3 days. In situations of poor absorption and diarrhoea occurring this time can be very short and in constipation it may be much longer.

Fate of nutrients in the body

Once absorbed into the blood stream the nutrients are available for various metabolic processes in the body.

The carbohydrates which have been absorbed as glucose into the bloodstream pass around the body.

FATE OF NUTRIENTS

- **Carbohydrates**
  - **Pass in bloodstream directly to liver**
  - **Carried in blood to cells in body**
  - **Converted to glycogen**
  - **Converted to fats**

- **Fats**
  - **Fatty acids rebuilt to triglycerides**
  - **Fatty acids released, used for energy**

- **Proteins**
  - **Amino acids for use in reforming body proteins, enzymes, hormones**
  - **Converted into non-essential amino acids**
  - **Oxidised for energy**
  - **Proteins cannot be stored**

They can be:

1. taken up by all cells of the body for use as energy. For cells to take up glucose from the blood stream they require the hormone insulin, which is secreted by the pancreas;
2. converted into glycogen for storage in the liver and muscles, as a short-term energy reserve; and
3. converted into body fat for storage in the adipose tissue (fat) of the body.

The proteins which have been absorbed as amino acids into the bloodstream pass around the body. They are first taken to the liver where they can be:

1. passed back into the blood stream as amino acids from which they can be taken up by the cells of the body for use in the production of structural cell proteins, hormones or enzymes;
2. converted by the liver into those amino acids which are in short supply. Only the non-essential amino acids can be made by the liver. Essential amino acids must be provided by the diet; and
3. converted by the liver into glucose which can then be used for energy or converted into body fat. This process occurs in the liver and is referred to as deamination whereby the amino acids have the nitrogen removed from the molecule and the remainder is converted into glucose. The waste nitrogen is converted into urea by the liver which is then excreted via the kidneys in the urine. Proteins cannot be stored by the body.

The fatty acids which have been absorbed into the bloodstream pass around the body. In the bloodstream the fatty acids are carried as triglycerides. After a fatty meal, because of all the fat as triglycerides, the blood has a milky appearance. The triglycerides can be:

1. taken up by all cells of the body for use as energy. On reaching the cells the triglycerides are broken down into fatty acids which are used for energy; and
2. converted into body fat for storage in the adipose tissue (fat) of the body. Dietary fat is easily converted into body fat which gives a constant source of energy.

Vitamins and Minerals

Water-soluble vitamins cannot be stored by the body but the fat-soluble ones can be stored in the liver. Proteins like water-soluble vitamins and minerals are not stored by the body.

Energy release

The body is a complex living structure composed of billions of individual cells, all of

---

ENERGY PROVIDED

The energy provided by carbohydrate, protein, alcohol and fat in food and drinks

1g carbohydrate provides 3.75kcal (16kJ)

1g protein provides 4kcal (17kJ)

1g alcohol provides 7kcal (29kJ)

1g of fat provides 9kcal (37kJ)

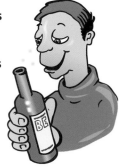

The micronutrients (vitamins and minerals), fibre and water do not provide energy

which require energy from foods to function and hence metabolism to occur.

The energy is derived from foods such as carbohydrates, proteins and fats. Alcohol also provides energy.

Basal Metabolic Rate (BMR)

Energy is required for all of the metabolic actions to occur in the body. These processes include the basic ones required to keep us alive and occur continuously. We are not aware of them; they are referred to as involuntary activities. They all require energy and the amount of energy required is called the Basal Metabolic Rate (BMR).

Energy requirements

Everyone needs energy from food to live. Energy is required for all of the vital functions of the body such as maintenance of the body temperature, breathing, digestion, blood circulation, hormone release and all of the other cellular activities that occur in the body. Energy is also needed for growth and repair of body tissues.

Energy is measured in both kilojoules and megajoules abbreviated as kJ and MJ respectively. Energy is also measured in kilocalories (kcal).

The simple way of converting energy in kilocalories to kilojoules is to multiply by 4.2.

The recommendations for the amount of energy needed for different individuals are called the Estimated Average Requirements (EAR) and are found in the publication entitled 'Reference Nutrient Intakes for the UK'.

The EAR varies according to the age and gender of the individual. In general, males aged 15-18 years have the highest energy requirements because of their activity level which tends to be high and also because they are still requiring energy for growth to occur.

During pregnancy a woman only requires an extra 200 kcal per day during the last trimester (the last third of pregnancy). During the period of lactation (breastfeeding) for the first month an extra 450 kcal per day are required, the second month an extra 530 kcal per day and for the third month an extra kcal per day. Therefore breastfeeding can produce a major demand for energy in the diet.

ENERGY REQUIREMENTS Estimated average requirements (EARs) kcal/day		
	Males	**Females**
0-3 months	545	515
4-6 months	690	645
7-9 months	825	765
10-12 months	920	865
1-3 years	1230	1165
4-6 years	1715	1545
7-10 years	1970	1740
11-14 years	2220	2110
15-18 years	2755	2110
19-50 years	2550	1940
51-59 years	2550	1900
60-64 years	2380	1900
65-74 years	2330	1900
75+ years	2100	1810

Activity has a profound effect on the energy requirements and therefore the energy requirements of very active individuals can be much greater than those of very inactive people. Today the lack of exercise is a major contributor to obesity as people do not perform enough exercise to burn up the amount of energy taken from food in the diet.

Different people need different amounts of energy.

In general women need less energy than men; this is because women tend to have a smaller body size and also be less active. Men also generally have a greater amount of muscle tissue than women.

As people age they tend to need less energy as they are usually less active. They also tend to have a smaller proportion of muscle tissue than younger people.

Active people need more energy than inactive ones. In general muscle tissue requires more energy for its metabolism than does adipose tissues. Hence sportspeople and very active individuals need more energy due to the amount of energy expended in the activity itself plus the energy requirements of the muscle tissue itself.

The recommendations for the average proportion of energy

- **33% of total energy should come from fat**

- **47% should come from carbohydrate foods**

- **Protein intake averages 15% of total energy intake**

- **Alcohol should contribute on average around 5% of energy intake**

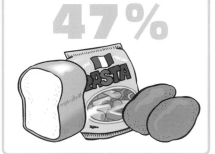

DIFFERENT NEEDS - DIFFERENT PEOPLE

- Gender
  - **Women tend to need less energy than men**

- Age
  - **Older adults need less energy than growing adolescents**

- Physical activity
  - **The more active a person is the greater their energy needs**

- Life events
  - **Such as pregnancy or illness change people's energy and nutrient needs**

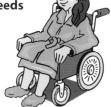

ENERGY USED
The average energy used with different activities

ACTIVITY	ENERGY USED IN 20 MINUTES
Sleeping	16 kcal
Reading	20 kcal
Driving	30 kcal
Walking	80 kcal
Swimming	110 kcal
Jogging	140 kcal
Running fast	200 kcal

Life events such as pregnancy and breastfeeding can increase the energy requirements. Illnesses where the body temperature is increased increase the energy requirements. Accidents or injuries where healing needs to occur also increase the energy requirements.

For health it is recommended that the major source of energy in the diet is from starchy carbohydrate foods.

Question to determine progress
What is digestion? What is absorption? **See answer in the appendix.**

7 Nutrition for different life stages

Introduction

Good nutrition is absolutely vital to all people no matter what their age. Nutrition affects the health and the day-to-day feelings of well-being for all and can have a profound effect on how elderly people feel and function. Also, for babies and children their growth and development and future health status are all dependent on essential nutrients, which they obtain from food.

Energy in the diet

The energy requirements vary according to the age and activity of the individual.

The normal proportions of energy in the diet are advocated as being:

1. 33-35% energy from fat
2. 47-50% energy from carbohydrate
3. 15% energy from protein.

However, these proportions are those recommended in the diet of healthy adults. For babies and children under five years of age and elderly people the proportion of energy from fat is often increased due to limitations in the appetite.

Babies

Breast milk is the ideal food for the growing infant. Babies grow rapidly during the first few months of life and breast milk provides all of the nutrients that a baby requires for health in this period. The milk provides about 700 kcal per day for the infant. Additionally breast milk provides a number of other advantages to the mother and child. They are as follows:

	ESTIMATED AVERAGE REQUIREMENTS FOR ENERGY	
Age	Males kcal/day	Females kcal/day
0-3 months	545	515
4-6 months	690	645
7-9 months	825	765
10-12 months	920	865
1-3 years	1230	1165
4-6 years	1715	1545
7-10 years	1970	1740
11-14 years	2220	1845
15-18 years	2755	2110
19-50 years	2550	1940
51-59 years	2550	1900
60-64 years	2380	1900
65-74 years	2330	1900
75+ years	2100	1810

Pregnancy 3rd trimester extra 200 kcal per day
Lactating 1st month extra 450 kcal per day
Lactating 2nd month extra 530 kcal per day
Lactating 3rd month extra 570 kcal per day
Lactating 4th–6th months extra 480 kcal per day

- it enables the mother to regain her pre-pregnancy figure easily and to lose any extra weight gained in pregnancy;
- it contains all nutrients in the correct amount needed for the growing baby. Breast milk is low in iron and copper but infants have a store of this in the body which lasts for the first few months of life;

- it is the correct temperature;
- it is sterile; this is particularly important in underdeveloped countries where there are poor sources of clean water;
- it contains antibodies which confer advantages to the child in resisting infections and diseases;
- it can help the mother-child bonding process;
- It cannot be over-concentrated; and
- it is particularly helpful for any infants where there is a history of allergies in the family.

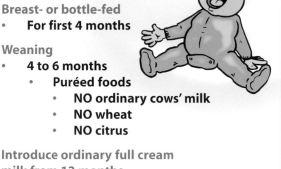

BABIES

- **Breast milk**
  - **Provides antibodies**

- **Breast- or bottle-fed**
  - **For first 4 months**

- **Weaning**
  - **4 to 6 months**
    - **Puréed foods**
      - **NO ordinary cows' milk**
      - **NO wheat**
      - **NO citrus**

- **Introduce ordinary full cream milk from 12 months**

If the mother is unable to breast-feed then an infant-formula milk can be used. These formulas are made from cows' milk which is adapted to provide a composition as similar as possible to breast milk. These formulae must be correctly made up as If they are over-concentrated they can put an excessive load on the babies' developing kidneys.

In hot weather it is important that babies are given extra fluid.

It has recently been recommended that babies are exclusively breast- or bottle-fed for the first six months of life.

Weaning

Solid foods (which are in a smooth, puréed or liquidised form) are given to a baby in the process of weaning. Such foods are given from the age of 4-6 months.

It is recommended that the first foods given to a baby are baby rice, puréed potatoes or other vegetables. A spoonful is usually introduced before either breast or infant milk feeds. The puréed foods can be home-made or commercial ones.

As the iron stores that a baby is born with only last for about the first 4-6 months of life, it is important that a good source of iron such as red meat is introduced into the infant's diet.

To prevent early allergies occurring it is recommended that before six months of age the foods more likely to cause problems are not given. These include:

- citrus fruits;
- wheat and wheat-containing foods; and
- products containing nuts.

Other foods such as those containing a lot of sugar or those containing a lot of additives, including artificial sweeteners, are also not advised.

Gradually the amounts of solids are increased and also the texture made lumpier as the child develops teeth. During the teething stage, hard items such as rusks or pieces of hard vegetable such as carrots are useful for the child to chew on under supervision to ensure no choking occurs.

By one year of age a child should be eating a varied diet. It is not recommended that ordinary cows' milk is given to infants before one year of age but infant formula milk should be continued until then.

Pre-school children

A varied diet should be continued for pre-school children without the addition of foods containing high levels of sugar or salt.

Sugar and sugary drinks provided between meals have been linked with dental decay (dental caries). Sugar promotes the growth of bacteria in the mouth and these produce acids, which erode the teeth. If children are given sugary sweets, (and sweets and sugar are not needed by children for healthy diet) the best time for them to be eaten is at the end of a meal.

Children between 1 and 3 years are prone to iron deficiency anaemia which can be due to inadequate amounts of iron in the diet. Therefore it is important that young children are given a good source of dietary iron such as red meat or, if vegetarian, a good range of iron-containing foods such as peas, beans and lentils.

Young children may choke on items such as nuts, boiled sweets and gobstoppers, and therefore these should not be given to pre-school children.

Full cream milk should be given to young children. Semi-skimmed milk can be introduced at two years of age and fully skimmed milk at age five years.

School-age children

Children of this age are growing very fast and are also usually very active. The energy requirements for a girl aged 7-10 years are similar to those for an adult woman. Thiamin requirements are also high as this vitamin is needed for energy metabolism.

There is usually a growth spurt in children just before the onset of puberty (ages 11-13 years). It is important to offer children a varied diet with plenty of energy from large portions of starchy carbohydrates, plenty of fruit and vegetables and a good source of calcium and protein from milk and milk-containing foods.

Dental health is important and a diet without excessive sugar consumption is recommended.

Children also need a high intake of calcium due to skeletal growth. This can be provided by milk, cheese and fish with small bones. Nowadays children often drink more soft drinks than milk.

Adolescents

The nutritional needs of adolescents are higher in most respects than for any other age group because of the growth and activity that occur. Adolescents usually go through the end of a growth spurt with extra requirements for energy, calcium and protein.

Today, young people are very definite in their views on nutrition and what they will eat.

CHILDREN

• **Growing fast and very active**

• **Energy requirements for 7-10 year-old girl and need for thiamin nearly as high as an adult woman**

• **Calcium – milk**

• **Dental health:**
  • **sensible eating habits**
  • **avoid sugary snacks**
  • **clean teeth**

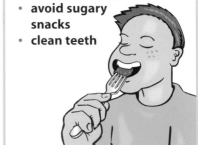

Indeed the food choice of children is an area where they begin to demonstrate independence from their parents which is particularly striking during the adolescent years. Appetising meals, which are easy to eat and which provide a good balance of nutrients, are vital for the health and well-being of youngsters. Not only does good food bring satisfaction and pleasure but also for young people it maintains their current nutritional status and has a major impact on their future health and well-being. Thus good nutrition can play a role in maximising their health, activity, cognitive ability and helping to prevent the onset of future health problems.

Bone health is related to adequate calcium and vitamin D during the growing years. Young people derive most of their requirements for vitamin D by the action of sunlight on their skin. Those who do not eat meat or oily fish, or do not go out of doors or who wear clothing that fully covers them, need to take a dietary source of vitamin D.

The Department of Health and Ministry of Agriculture, Fisheries and Food (DEFRA) carried out a survey of the diet of people aged from 4 to 18 years. This showed that young people were not eating enough fruit and vegetables and took too much saturated fat and salt. Of particular concern is the fact that about 50% of teenage girls were not taking enough iron and 20% were not taking enough calcium. The main foods eaten by the children surveyed were white bread, savoury snacks, potato chips, biscuits, mashed potatoes, jacket potatoes and chocolate.

As regards alcohol, the survey showed that 44% of young men and 43% of young women aged 15 years had consumed alcohol in the week prior to interview. The study also found that an average of 13% of boys and 14% of girls were regular smokers. Smoking has implications for the vitamin C content of the diet. It is recommended that an intake of up to 80 mg of vitamin C per day is needed for smokers. As already shown young people are taking too little fruit and vegetables, the major sources of vitamin C in the diet. This could have worrying consequences for the future as regards incidence of heart disease and cancers.

The survey of the health of young people showed 30% of 16-20 year olds were judged to be overweight or obese, which can obviously contribute to the development of future health problems.

The diet and lifestyle of teenage girls may be of particular concern, as they were shown to have a diet low in calcium and iron. They also take too much saturated fat and too little fruit and vegetables. Additionally, as already mentioned, a worrying proportion of this group tends to take excessive amounts of alcohol and smoke cigarettes. Of particular concern among teenage girls is that only 13% of them take moderate exercise on five or more days per week.

TEENAGERS

- Iron
  - required for formation of haemoglobin

- Calcium & Vitamin D
  - **45% of adult skeleton laid down in adolescence**

- Folate
  - **pregnancy increased requirement**

DIETARY REQUIREMENTS FOR NUTRIENTS FOR GROWING YOUNG PEOPLE

As can be seen, the dietary reference values for young people are high during the teenage years. Iron is particularly required by teenage girls, when a monthly blood loss occurs. Zinc is important in teenage boys for male fertility.

DIETARY REFERENCE VALUES FOR GIRLS AGED 11– 18 YEARS

	Units	Age (years)	
		11-14	15-18
Energy	MJ	7.92	8.83
	Kcal	1845	2110
Protein	g	41.2	45.0
Iron	mg	14.8	14.8
Calcium	mg	800	800
Zinc	mg	9.0	7.0
Magnesium	mg	280	300
Phosphorus	mg	625	625
Sodium	mg	1600	1600
Vitamin A	µg	600	600
Vitamin B$_1$, thiamin	mg	0.7	0.8
Vitamin B$_2$, riboflavin	mg	1.1	1.1
Niacin	mg	12	14
Vitamin B$_6$	mg	1.0	1.2
Vitamin B$_{11}$	µg	1.2	1.5
Folate	µg	200	200
Vitamin C	mg	35	40

DIETARY REFERENCE VALUES FOR BOYS AGED 11– 18 YEARS

	Units	Age (years)	
		11-14	15-18
Energy	MJ	9.27	11.51
	Kcal	2200	2755
Protein	g	42.1	55.2
Iron	mg	11.3	11.3
Calcium	mg	1000	1000
Zinc	mg	9.0	9.5
Magnesium	mg	280	300
Phosphorus	mg	775	775
Sodium	mg	1600	1600
Vitamin A	µg	600	700
Vitamin B$_1$, thiamin	mg	0.9	1.1
Vitamin B$_2$, riboflavin	mg	1.2	1.3
Niacin	mg	15	18
Vitamin B$_6$	mg	1.2	1.5
Vitamin B$_{12}$	µg	1.2	1.5
Folate	µg	200	200
Vitamin C	mg	35	40

This is in comparison with 70% of girls aged 5 years and 29% of teenage boys. Again this can have detrimental effects on their weight and future health.

Teenage girls are the group that are most affected by anorexia nervosa as well as having concerns regarding being overweight and trying to follow inappropriate diets. Finally this group of teenage girls is the one which may have early pregnancies with the demands that makes on the diet.

School meals

Free school meals were first provided in the 1860s to poor school children in London.

In 1944 the Education Act stipulated that local authorities must provide a school meal of a nutritional standard, ie to provide a third of the current nutritional requirements for children per meal. This situation continued until 1980 when the Education Act was changed and local authorities were no longer required to provide school meals except for those entitled to free ones. There were no nutritional standards for the meals that were provided and schools were free to provide school meals of whatever composition they wanted.

New nutritional standards for school lunches

The Government published the Nutritional Standards for School Lunches (Department for Education and Employment, 2000).

The Nutritional Standards for School Lunches are based on the five food groups shown in the Balance of Good Health, which is the National Food Guide for nutritional education. The five food groups are:

A. **Fruit and vegetables**
   Includes all fruit and vegetables in all forms whether fresh, frozen, canned or as juices.
B. **Starchy foods**
   Includes bread, chappatis, pasta, noodles, rice, potatoes, sweet potatoes, yam, millet and cornmeal.
C. **Meat, fish and other non-dairy sources of protein**
   Including eggs, nuts, pulses and beans except green beans. These items can be fresh, frozen, dried or canned.
D. **Milk and dairy foods**
   Includes cheese, yoghurt, fromage frais and custards but not butter or cream.
E. **Foods containing fat and foods containing sugar**
   Includes margarine, mayonnaise, cream, chocolate, cakes and pastries.

The requirements are varied according to the needs of the age group of children.

Nutritional requirements for children who attend nursery schools or nursery units in primary schools are as follows:
   ◆   food from each of the groups A, B, C and D should be available each day;
   ◆   particular emphasis was put on group A;
   ◆   fresh fruit, fruit tinned in juice or fruit should be available every day;
   ◆   a fruit-based dessert should be available at least twice a week; and
   ◆   a type of vegetable (not from group B) should be available every day.

Within group B, fat or oil should not be used in the cooking process on more than three days per week.

Within group C, fish should be available on at least one day per week and red meat on at least two days per week.

Nutritional requirements for pupils at secondary schools

Two types of food from each of groups A, B, C and D should be available each day.
In group A, both a fruit and vegetable should be available.
Within group B on every day, a food that is not cooked in fat or oil should be available.
Within group C, fish should be available on at least two days per week and red meat on at least three days per week.

Breakfast eating

Breakfast has long been recognised as an important meal. It is vital not from just a nutritional view but in the way it enhances cognitive performance and hence the ability of children to learn. Initiatives such as 'breakfast clubs' have been incorporated into some schools.

Women

Adult women need to have a well-balanced and varied diet without excessive amounts of energy and fat to prevent obesity developing. For the average woman a diet providing about 30% of the energy from fat would contain about 70g of fat.

Iron is important in a woman's diet to meet the needs of the body and to counteract the monthly blood loss. The iron requirements for women are greater than those of men.

Calcium is also important in a woman's diet to maintain the bone structure of the skeleton.

For any woman contemplating becoming pregnant or who is pregnant, a supplement of folic acid should be taken. Normally 400 micrograms of folic acid is recommended each day for the first 12 weeks of pregnancy. This helps to prevent neural tube defects such as spina bifida.

The foetus is completely dependent on the mother for providing the essential nutrients. Nutrients and oxygen pass from the mother's bloodstream to the foetus via the placenta.

It is important during pregnancy that the mother does not 'eat for two' and gain excessive amounts of weight, which may be difficult to lose after the baby is born. Some extra weight gain is useful during pregnancy as an insurance against the energy needs of the woman for breastfeeding.

It is during the 3rd trimester, which

PREGNANCY AND BREASTFEEDING

- **Iron, calcium and folate (folic acid)**

- **Food poisoning (e.g. salmonellosis) can increase the risk of miscarriage**

- **A number of foods should be restricted or avoided during pregnancy**
    - **Liver and liver-containing foods (e.g. liver pâté) because of their potentially high vitamin A content**
    - **Foods which increase the risk of food-borne infections e.g. listeria poisoning**

WOMEN
• **Approx 70g fat per day maximum for average woman taking 2000 calories (30% from fat)**
• **Folic acid**
• **Iron**
• **Calcium**
• **Energy intake to balance output**
• **Fluid**

is the last third of pregnancy, that energy requirements are increased, but only by 200 kcal per day.

It is important that the mother's diet contains sufficient protein, iron, calcium and vitamins to sustain both the needs of the mother and also the development of the foetus. During pregnancy, weight gain occurs as the foetus develops, the uterus (womb) also develops, blood volume increases and breast tissues enlarge.

During the period of breastfeeding the mother's calorie requirements, and those for protein, calcium, phosphorus, magnesium, zinc, copper and selenium as well as the B vitamins, vitamin C, vitamin A and D are all increased to enable the mother to produce breast milk.

During pregnancy high levels of vitamin A can have an adverse effect on the foetus. For this reason, supplements containing vitamin A are not recommended. Also liver and foods containing it such as pâté are not recommended due to the high levels of vitamin A they contain.

Also pregnant women and the foetus are more susceptible to foodborne infections such as listeria which is found in soft cheeses made from unpasteurised milk, unwashed vegetables and chilled foods.

Food poisoning bacteria such as salmonella can increase the risk of miscarriage, so good food hygiene should be practised and any foods such as raw eggs avoided in dishes like mousses and mayonnaises.

Men

Men have a higher energy requirement than women due to them having a general higher activity level than women and also a greater muscle mass in the body.

Men require more zinc than women for sexual functioning.

Coronary heart disease is more common in men than women and therefore it is important that men avoid this by watching the amount of saturated fat in their diet, ensuring that they take plenty of fruit and vegetables and avoid becoming obese.

Many men become obese because of a lifestyle with too little exercise and too many calories, which can often be derived from fat and excess alcohol.

Elderly people

Elderly people vary a great deal in their activity levels, nutritional status and health. In general, as people age, various processes occur which can have an impact on their nutritional status:

1. decreased muscle mass, which causes less muscle strength;
2. decreased immune function, making them more prone to illnesses and infections;

MEN
• **Larger muscles**
• **Larger liver**
• **Require more zinc**
• **Activity**
• **Coronary heart disease**
• **Obesity**

3. decreased organ function, leading to problems such as constipation;
4. decreased nutrient absorption, leading to a reduced iron and zinc absorption;
5. decreased hormone production, leading to the development of disorders such as type 2 diabetes as the production of insulin occurs;
6. decreased taste, smell and vision, thus making food less tempting to eat;
7. decreased appetite, resulting in a poor nutritional reduces;
8. decreased mobility and flexibility, which can make shopping, cooking and eating difficult;
9. decreased thirst response, which means that too little fluid is consumed which contributes to dehydration with resultant bowel and kidney disorders and confusion;
10. increased bone loss – osteoporosis affects one in five women over 50 years of age. The resultant thinning of bones causes pain and also makes fractures more common;
11. dental problems, causing difficulties in eating;
12. lower incomes, meaning it is difficult to afford a balanced diet; and
13. loneliness, which can be due to the loss of a partner and can mean food becomes neglected.

Those living in their own homes are more likely to be better nourished than those living in institutions.

It is important that to maintain health in elderly people the diet is adequate in:
♦ energy, to maintain activity levels;
♦ protein to maintain body tissues;
♦ vitamin C to promote the functioning of the immune system;
♦ calcium and vitamin D to maintain the bone structure. Most people get enough vitamin D by the action of sunlight on their skin but elderly people may not go out of doors or expose their skin to sunlight and thus need a source of vitamin D in the diet. This can be derived from margarine, full cream milk and oily fish;
♦ iron such as from red meat. Anaemia due to a lack of dietary iron and a decreased absorption of iron from foods is a problem in elderly people. The symptoms of iron deficiency anaemia are tiredness and apathy, which can exacerbate an elderly person's lack of interest in food;

ELDERLY PEOPLE

• **Many older people do not have enough vitamin D in their diet, which is necessary for bone health**

• **Some older people have low intakes of some vitamins (e.g. folate and vitamin C) and minerals (e.g. magnesium, potassium and zinc)**

• **Those without their own teeth, living in institutions or from lower socio-economic groups, are at the highest risk of vitamin and mineral deficiencies**

- plenty of dietary fibre (NSP) from fruit and vegetables and high-fibre breakfast cereals and wholemeal bread can help to keep the bowel functioning correctly and prevent constipation, which is a problem in many elderly people;
- adequate fluid (approximately two litres per day) ensures the correct functioning of the kidneys and digestive tract. It also helps to prevent problems such as cystitis from occurring;
- a good store cupboard of dry goods can prevent someone who is unwell or frail having to shop in bad weather;
- also a freezer and microwave can help those with difficulties in cooking from having to spend a long time preparing meals and give variety;
- delivered meals and supermarket deliveries ordered via the internet can also help people who have difficulty in obtaining food items; and
- luncheon clubs can encourage those who live on their own to eat in a social atmosphere.

Question to determine progress

Describe weaning and when it occurs. **See answer in the appendix.**

8 Healthy eating and malnutrition

Diet and health

Various health problems have been associated with a poor diet. However there are no unhealthy foods, only unbalanced and therefore unhealthy diets.

A healthy diet is one which:

♦ people enjoy eating and provides variety and enough energy and nutrients for health and well-being;

♦ provides plenty of starchy foods like bread, rice, pasta, potatoes, noodles;

♦ includes plenty of fruit and vegetables;

♦ does not contain excessive amounts of fat, particularly saturated fat;

♦ contains moderate amounts of milk and dairy products;

♦ contains moderate amounts of meat, fish or alternatives; and

♦ does not contain excessive quantities of sugary foods.

Malnutrition

The term malnutrition means unbalanced or disordered eating and results in adverse consequences to health. It is often considered in the context of underdeveloped countries and the situation of starvation.

Under-nutrition

Malnutrition can take the form of 'under-nutrition' or 'over-nutrition'. Under-nutrition occurs mainly in underdeveloped countries where problems such as marasmus and kwashiorkor, due to too little dietary energy or protein occur. Under-nutrition can occur in developed countries due to an unbalanced diet with problems such as anaemia developing due to too little dietary iron.

Over-nutrition

This is more likely to occur in developed countries with over-consumption of energy from food resulting in obesity, excess saturated fat contributing to coronary heart disease, excess salt contributing to high blood pressure, excessive consumption of alcohol leading to liver cirrhosis and frequent consumption of sugar contributing to dental caries (tooth decay).

MALNUTRITION
• **Under-nutrition**
• **Scurvy**
• **Anaemias of different types**
• **Beriberi**
• **Diverticular disease**
• **Starvation**
• **Rickets**
• **Osteomalacia**
• **Failure to thrive**
• **Over-nutrition**
• **Obesity**
• **Type 2 diabetes**
• **Dental caries**
• **Coronary heart disease**
• **Hypertension**
• **Liver disorders**

Currently in the UK:

♦ over half the adult population is overweight;

♦ 400 people die from coronary heart disease each day;

♦ cancer affects 1 in 3 people and causes 25% of all deaths;

♦ over 1 million people have been diagnosed with diabetes; and

♦　2 in 5 men and 1 in 3 women have high blood pressure.

DISORDERS RELATING TO OVER-NUTRITION

Obesity

More than 60% of men and more than 50% of women are overweight. This is because the amount of energy (calories) consumed is too high in relation to levels of physical activity. Being very overweight increases the risk of a number of diseases, including heart disease, stroke, diabetes and some types of cancer.

Obesity can be measured by various means, such as:

♦　weighing individuals with scales and comparing the weight with height-weight charts;

♦　assessing the body mass index (BMI). This is the relationship between height and weight as assessed by the formula whereby the weight in kilograms is divided by the height in metres squared.
The resultant BMI is a number usually between 15 and 50. Research has shown that this number gives an assessment of the health risk for an individual according to their weight in relationship to their height.

WAYS OF MEASURING OBESITY
• **Height-weight tables**
• **Body mass index**
• **Waist-hip ratios**
• **Waist measurements**
• **Skinfold measurements**

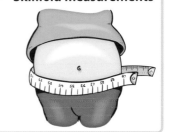

♦　A BMI below 20 signifies someone who is underweight and who can have health risks in relationship to this.

♦　A BMI between 20 and 25 is in the normal weight range at which there are few health risks.

♦　A BMI of 26 to 30 indicates someone is overweight. While this carries few health risks it is easy for someone to continue to gain weight and thus become obese.

♦　A BMI of over 30 is considered to be indicative of obesity with numerous health risks.

♦　A BMI of over 40 is considered to be indicative of severe obesity and is strongly associated with severe health problems.

♦　To save doing calculations, BMI charts are often used to calculate the BMI.

♦　waist-hip ratios are used in measuring obesity using a tape measure. The most unhealthy area for the weight to be carried is around the waist and stomach area. This is called 'central obesity' or an 'apple shape' and is found more frequently in men. Such a form of obesity is associated more frequently with heart disease, type 2 diabetes and high blood pressure than being a 'pear shape' with extra fat distributed on the hips and legs as is more common in women. The ratio between the measurement of hips and waist should be large;

♦　waist measurements alone are also often used to assess the level of obesity. Generally men should have a waist measurement of below 94 cm (37 inches) and women 80 cm (31 inches);

♦　skinfold calipers can be used to assess body fat levels by measuring the deposition of fat below the skin in various areas of the body; and

♦ electrical impedance methods can also be used to assess the percentage of body fat. This method requires a special measurement tool.

Problems associated with obesity

Numerous problems are associated with obesity.

Type 2 diabetes

Diabetes is due to the body being unable to produce adequate amounts of the hormone effective insulin.

Insulin is produced by the pancreas and is required to enable cells of the body to take up glucose, which is circulating in the blood for energy. Without insulin the glucose level in the blood rises and eventually spills over into the urine, due to the kidney being unable to retain high levels. The symptoms of diabetes are usually excessive thirst and frequent passing of urine.

Diabetes can result in complications such as visual problems, peripheral nerve problems causing a lack of sensitivity in feet, a feeling of being constantly tired, an increased risk of heart disease and kidney disorders. Good control of the diabetes helps to reduce the onset of these complications. Diabetes is usually regularly monitored by measurements of weight, blood pressure , blood sugar levels and examinations of the eyes and feet.

> ## PROBLEMS ASSOCIATED WITH OBESITY
>
> - **Heart disease**
> - **Hypertension**
> - **Joint problems**
> - **Breathlessness**
> - **Type 2 diabetes**
> - **Strokes**
> - **Varicose veins**
> - **Accidents**
> - **Certain cancers**
> - **Poor recovery from surgery**
> - **Psychological problems**
> - **Social problems**

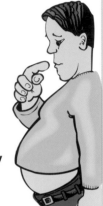

There are 2 types of diabetes:

Type 1 which requires insulin for treatment. This type of diabetes particularly is diagnosed in young people of normal weight and requires insulin for its control. The initial symptoms of diabetes are severe and the onset is rapid.

Type 2 diabetes occurs in overweight people. It is controlled by diet and possibly tablets. It is important that the overweight person with type 2 diabetes loses weight as the fat cells in the adipose tissue are resistant to the action of insulin. The symptoms are usually mild and may remain undetected for years.

The most common type of diabetes is type 2 and weight loss can enable the sufferer to achieve normal blood glucose levels, cease any loss of glucose in the urine, reduce the risk of complications and enhance the feeling of well-being.

Cancer

Every year, 32,000 people in the UK die of cancer before they reach their 65th birthday. It is estimated that a poor diet contributes to around a quarter of all cancers. In particular, low consumption of fruit and vegetables is linked with an increased risk of bowel (colorectal) and stomach cancer (and possibly some other cancers). Breast cancer is linked with obesity. Cancer treatment costs the NHS £1.3 billion per year.

FRUIT AND VEGETABLES

- **5 portions of fruit and vegetables may protect against chronic diseases, such as cancer and heart disease**

- **A portion of fruit or vegetables means:**
    - **Half a large fruit (e.g. avocado, grapefruit)**
    - **1 medium sized vegetable or fruit (e.g. apple, pear, banana)**
    - **2 small fruits (e.g plums)**
    - **1 cup of small fruits (e.g. grapes)**
    - **A tablespoon of dried fruits (e.g. dates)**
    - **2-3 tablespoons cooked or canned fruit**
    - **2 tablespoons cooked, frozen or canned vegetables**
    - **A bowl of salad**
    - **A glass of fruit juice (one per day)**

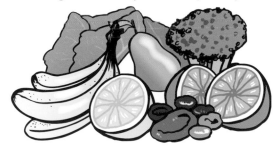

Cancer is linked with a number of dietary factors including obesity, excessive quantities of fat in the diet, too little dietary fibre (NSP) and too few antioxidants.

The inclusion of plenty of fruit and vegetables in the diet appears to have a protective effect due to the antioxidant content of fruit and vegetables.

It is recommended that 400g, (approximately 1lb) of fruit and vegetables are taken each day. This is usually interpreted as five portions of fruit and vegetables per day.

Coronary heart disease (CHD)

The UK has one of the highest rates of heart disease in western Europe. Every year, 25,000 people die of heart disease, stroke and related illnesses before they reach their 65th birthday. A diet containing too much fat, salt and not enough fruit and vegetables is an important contributing factor to the risk of heart disease, certain cancers and stroke. A diet high in saturated fat, for example, raises cholesterol levels in the blood. Obesity also contributes to CHD and fruit and vegetables appear to have a preventative effect.

Reducing the amount of all fat in the diet has been recommended, but the type of fat is also important. The fatty acid composition of fats not only affects their cooking qualities and storage properties, it also contributes to people's health.

All fats contain a mixture of different fatty acids but choosing those which contain higher amounts of unsaturates (polyunsaturates or monounsaturates), rather than saturates, is preferable.

Again it is recommended that fruit and vegetables are taken as part of the diet.

High blood pressure (Hypertension)

Too much salt (sodium chloride) is linked to high blood pressure. Having a high blood pressure or blood cholesterol level substantially increases the chances of suffering from heart disease or a stroke.

Reducing the average daily salt intake by a third could cut deaths from heart disease by 22% and from stroke by 16%, saving 34,000 lives a year.

At present we take an average of 9g of salt per person per day. Salt is made up of sodium and chloride with about 1g of sodium being found in 2.5g of salt. Sodium is the component of salt that has a harmful effect on blood pressure. Salt is particularly found in manufactured foods such as canned soups, canned vegetables and meals. It is also found in savoury snacks such as potato crisps and salted peanuts, and items such as cheese, bacon and ham. Salted fish contain salt where it is used as a preservative.

Sodium is also found in monosodium glutamate which is used as a flavour enhancer in manufactured foods such as chilled and frozen meals.

Some people take sodium bicarbonate as an antacid for stomach conditions and this will also contribute to the sodium intake.

Heart disease and stroke and related illnesses cost the NHS an estimated £3.8 billion a year

Dental Caries

Diet and dental caries (tooth decay) are strongly interlinked. Frequent consumption of sugar and foods containing sugar can cause the formation of plaques which are areas on the tooth containing bacteria and food debris. The bacteria produce acid which erodes the tooth causing decay to occur.

If sugary foods are chosen in preference to sugar free ones, they are best consumed at mealtimes to limit the effect on dental health.

Frequent consumption of acidic items such as fruit juices can also have a harmful effect on teeth.

Fluoride confers protection to teeth by making the enamel which covers the teeth be more resistant to attack by acids.

Liver cirrhosis

One of the major forms of liver disease is liver cirrhosis. This condition is associated with frequent over-consumption of alcohol.

The alcohol is normally detoxified by the liver but over-consumption causes the destruction of the liver cells.

SALT (SODIUM)

- **Salt as sodium chloride (1g of sodium is equivalent to around 2.5g of salt)**

- **Some foods labelled with the amount of sodium they contain in grams per 100g of the product**

- **Sodium in monosodium glutamate, sodium bicarbonate**

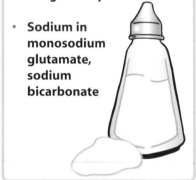

ALCOHOL

• **Beer/lager/cider**	**3-6% alcohol**
• **Wines**	**9-13% alcohol**
• **Spirits**	**37-45% alcohol**
• **Liqueurs**	**20-40% alcohol**
• **Fortified wines**	**18-25% alcohol**

- **Absorbed in stomach**
- **Broken down in liver**
- **7 calories per gram**

- **Unit of alcohol = 8 grams**
  - **Half pint of beer/lager/cider (300ml)**
  - **Glass of wine (100ml)**
  - **Tot of spirits (25ml)**

- **Upper safe limit**
  - **Men – 28 units per week**
  - **Women – 21 units per week**
  - **Alcohol-FREE day each week**

Often the over-consumption of alcohol is due to an addiction.

Alcohol is absorbed in the stomach where an excess can cause an irritation of the stomach lining resulting in gastritis.

The amount of alcohol in various alcoholic beverages varies. Spirits and liqueurs are the most concentrated forms of alcoholic beverages.

A unit of alcohol is considered to be a beverage containing 8g alcohol. Women are recommended to take no more than 21 units per week and men no more than 28 units per week.

Bulimia

The condition of bulimia nervosa is an eating disorder found in women in the age range 15-35 years. It is characterised by an urge to overeat, and sufferers may secretly consume large quantities of food. This over-consumption of vast amounts of food is counteracted by the sufferer vomiting and possibly taking large amounts of laxatives.

Peripheral nerve problems

Some individuals who take excessive amounts of vitamin B_6 may suffer from peripheral nerve problems causing a tingling in the fingers. This condition ceases when the supplement is ceased. The supplement is usually taken by women to treat symptoms of premenstrual syndrome.

This illustrates that over-consumption of vitamin supplements can be harmful to health.

DISORDERS RELATING TO UNDER-NUTRITION

Scurvy

This is due to lack of vitamin C which causes the blood vessels to break down and bleeding to occur into the joints. It used to be a cause of death in such people as sailors whose diet was deficient in vitamin C during their long voyages.

The diet of elderly people may be deficient in vitamin C and they can be easily prone to bruising because of this.

Anaemia

Anaemia can be due to a lack of iron in the diet. Iron is required for the formation of haemoglobin, which is found in the red blood cells. This substance carries oxygen from the lungs all around the body in the blood stream to the cells which use it in the energy release processes that occur.

A lack of iron in the diet means that insufficient haemoglobin is formed. As

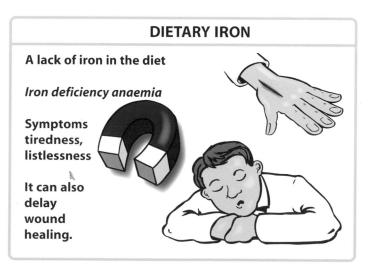

DIETARY IRON

A lack of iron in the diet

Iron deficiency anaemia

Symptoms tiredness, listlessness

It can also delay wound healing.

red blood cells last for only 120 days there needs to be a regular supply of dietary iron.

Symptoms of iron deficiency anaemia are tiredness, listlessness and delayed wound healing.

Those who have lost a lot of blood due to wounds, illness, or regular heavy periods or several pregnancies are particularly prone to iron deficiency anaemia. Infants about 18 months old and elderly people are also prone to anaemia. Those who do not take meat are also at risk unless they carefully maintain the amount of iron in the diet from vegetable sources.

Some people suffer from the form of anaemia called macrocytic anaemia caused by a deficiency of vitamin B_{12}. In this type of anaemia the red blood cells do not correctly develop. The symptoms are similar to those of iron deficiency anaemia.

Vitamin B_{12} is found in foods of animal origin such as meat, milk, fish and eggs and foods containing them. Those who are vegan may be at particular risk and need to ensure that adequate vitamin B_{12} is taken either from such products as yeast or from supplements.

Beriberi

This is due to a severe and prolonged lack of thiamin (vitamin B_1). It is seen in underdeveloped countries where the diet may be deficient in this vitamin.

It is sometimes seen in this country in alcoholics whose diet is predominated by alcohol and little other food.

Diverticular disease

This disorder is due to a lack of fluid and fibre in the diet. The wall of the colon or large intestine is usually smooth. When the diet lacks in fibre then the bowel may strain to pass waste products along it. In such situations the straining may cause diverticulae which are like small pockets to develop in the wall of the colon. These can cause pain as infections and waste products can remain in the diverticulae.

A high-fibre diet prevents the development of diverticulae or, if once developed, to prevent more developing and also to keep the existing ones infection-free.

Anorexia

Anorexia nervosa is a psychological eating disorder. It results in a refusal to eat (especially high calorie foods) and subsequent weight loss. Sometimes the desire of the sufferer to be slim may cause them to have a distorted body image whereby they consider they appear fatter than they actually are. It mainly affects girls but some boys are also affected. It is particularly prevalent in teenagers. Psychological treatment is usually required.

Rickets and osteomalacia

Most of the skeleton is deposited during the growing years especially during the teenage period. The deposition of calcium in the skeleton is called mineralisation and is balanced by demineralisation whereby calcium is lost from the bones.

Due to lack of vitamin D during childhood or the teenage years the condition of rickets can develop. Vitamin D assists the body to absorb calcium and without sufficient calcium the bones are not correctly mineralised and the bones become thin and weak. Due to this weakness the legs can become bowed in toddlers or knock knees can develop in teenagers.

Osteomalacia is the adult equivalent of rickets and is associated with bone demineralisation due to inadequate amounts of calcium and vitamin D.

BONE HEALTH PROBLEMS

- Rickets (toddlers and teenagers)
  - **Lack of vitamin D**
  - **Thin bones, bowed legs and knock knees**
  - **Asian children**

- Osteomalacia
  - **Adult equivalent of rickets**
  - **Bone demineralisation**

- Osteoporosis
  - **Number of factors – bone development in teenage years important**
  - **Hormonal effect – oestrogen in women and testosterone in men**
  - **Activity**
  - **Smoking**
  - **Alcohol**
  - **Balance of diet**
  - **Medication**

Osteoporosis is also associated with demineralisation due to advancing age. It occurs due to the loss of hormones such as the oestrogens which cease to be secreted after the menopause.

Various factors can contribute to osteoporosis such as:

- a diet poor in calcium and lack of activity can cause the skeleton to be poorly developed;
- some medications such as steroids can adversely affect calcium metabolism; and
- smoking and alcohol also affect calcium metabolism.

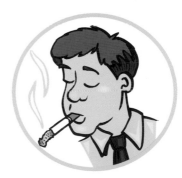

BASIS OF EATING FOR HEALTH

The Balance of Good Health

The national food guide is called the 'Balance of Good Health'; it is a diagram of a plate model upon which there are segments representing a healthy balanced diet.

The segments include:

- fruit and vegetables;
- bread, other cereals and potatoes;
- meat, fish and alternatives;
- milk and dairy foods; and
- foods containing fat and foods containing sugar.

The plate model is promoted by the Food Standards Agency as the one to be used for nutritional education and promotion in Great Britain. Therefore

THE BALANCE OF GOOD HEALTH

Fruit and vegetables

Bread, other cereals and potatoes

Meat, fish and alternatives

Foods containing fat Foods containing sugar

Milk and dairy foods

one often sees the model displayed in health promotion clinics and dining rooms as well as numerous booklets on nutrition and health.

While for those who are ill in hospital and for children the model may be adapted to give a greater proportion of calories and protein to assist recovery, it does give a useful way of looking at the different food and nutrient groups.

FRUIT AND VEGETABLES GROUP

The fruit and vegetables group includes all types of fruit and vegetables but excludes potatoes, which are considered to be a part of the group containing bread, other cereals and potatoes. Plantains or green bananas are also regarded as starchy carbohydrates and are therefore considered to be also part of the group containing potatoes.

Potatoes can be served as part of a dish such as shepherd's pie, curries and salads or as accompaniments. Potatoes can be mashed, baked, boiled, roast or chipped.

Vegetables such as pulses, i.e. dried or canned vegetables such as peas, beans and lentils, are considered to be a part of the meat, fish and alternative group. Pulses contain a good amount of protein and iron and thus can provide an alternative to meat in the diet of vegetarians and vegans.

Fruit and vegetables should form the basis of all meals and thus an emphasis is put on these foods

These are low in fat and again can help to adjust the contribution of energy from fat:
 ♦ fruit and vegetables can be fresh, frozen or canned;
 ♦ aim to have five portions of fruit and vegetables (400g) per day;
 ♦ fruit can form the basis of many puddings such as crumbles, summer puddings, roulades and hot or cold fruit salads;
 ♦ fruit can be set into low sugar jellies;
 ♦ fruit can be made into juices and smoothies which are tasty;
 ♦ vegetables can be added to curries, casseroles, in wraps, sandwiches, in stir-fries, as pizza toppings as well as accompaniments; and
 ♦ salads can be served as an extra side dish to meals.

The National School Fruit Scheme

This scheme was announced by the Department of Health in 2000 to improve the consumption of fruit and vegetables by children. The National Diet and Nutrition Survey had highlighted that among 4-6 year olds the consumption of fruit and vegetables was particularly low.

The scheme is due to be fully operational by 2004 and will provide all 4-6 year olds in primary schools with a free piece of fruit on each school day. Evaluated pilots to develop the scheme began in Autumn 2000 and continued in 2001. As part of the programme, five local five-a-day pilot initiatives, focusing on deprived communities, were initiated and rolled out across the country during 2002.

Whilst this scheme applies to England, initiatives to encourage healthy eating among school children are being developed in other parts of the UK. A similar scheme is being piloted in Scotland in some primary schools providing a portion of fruit three times a week.

Fats in fruit and vegetables

With the notable exceptions of olives and avocado pears, all fruit and vegetables are low in fat. Indeed they all contain only a trace of fat and are therefore low in calories and can be a very useful part of a low-calorie or low-fat diet.

Portion sizes

It is recommended that we all eat five portions of fruit and vegetables per day, that is, fruit and vegetables combined and not five portions of fruit and five portions of vegetables.

These five portions are based on the World Health Organisation recommendation that we should eat 400g of fruit and vegetables each day for the health benefits they provide.

Unfortunately in this country despite being encouraged to have five portions of fruit and vegetables per day in fact on average we only take three portions.

Fruit and vegetables as sources of iron and protein

The inclusion of extra pulses such as lentils or butter beans can easily be added to casseroles, stir fries and all types of main courses. Lentils can be of great use as they can thicken such dishes as curries and stews. They also provide extra protein and iron to a dish. Protein is particularly important to those patients in hospital, as it is required for healing to occur. Some iron is also found in pulses and this can be important in maintaining haemoglobin levels and thus helping to prevent anaemia.

Dried fruit can be used in cakes, scones and puddings such as bread and butter pudding. Dried fruits are a good source of calories, fibre and iron.

While the iron in pulses and dried fruit is in a non-haem form and thus not well absorbed, it does make a valuable contribution to the diet, especially of vegetarians and vegans.

Fruit and vegetables contain vitamin C and this enhances the absorption of non-haem iron, so this can be a valuable way of boosting the availability of iron in the diet.

Vitamins in fruit and vegetables

Fruit and vegetables contain a range of vitamins.

Ascorbic acid or vitamin C is found in all types of fruit and vegetables. It is required for healing to occur and necessary for the integrity of connective tissue. It is also an important antioxidant vitamin and as such it helps the body to resist diseases and infections by maximising the functioning of the immune system.

Especially rich sources of vitamin C are citrus fruits such as oranges and grapefruit as well as berry fruits like blackberries. Vegetables are also good sources, especially green vegetables, peppers and tomatoes. Even potatoes contain vitamin C. Thus potatoes can make a substantial contribution to vitamin C in the diet.

To maximise the amount of vitamin C in vegetables, cook them in a minimum amount of water and keep them warm for a minimum amount of time.

Carotenoids such as beta-carotene are found in a range of orange coloured fruits and vegetables like the obvious one of carrots. Beta-carotene is also present in apricots, tomatoes and mangoes. Dark green vegetables such as broccoli also contain it.

Carotene is an oxidant and like vitamin C has a positive effect on enhancing the immune system. Beta-carotene is the precursor for vitamin A which means that it is converted into it in the body.

Retaining nutrients in fruit and vegetables

It is important to try and retain as many of the nutrients in fruit and vegetables as possible. The water soluble vitamins are easily destroyed by oxidation by air over a period, heat and will also be leached out into the cooking water. The following suggestions can help to retain vitamins:

- ♦ try to use vegetables that are fresh;
- ♦ frozen vegetables are a good source of vitamins as they are picked and frozen rapidly;
- ♦ prepare and cook vegetables just prior to eating;
- ♦ do not over cook vegetables;
- ♦ avoid keeping vegetables warm for long periods;
- ♦ do not add bicarbonate of soda to cooking water;
- ♦ cook vegetables in a minimum of water;
- ♦ use cooking methods such as steaming and micro-waving;
- ♦ do not chop salad vegetables finely;
- ♦ use the water that vegetables have been cooked in for soups and gravies; and
- ♦ try not to peel vegetables and potatoes.

BREAD, OTHER CEREALS AND CARBOHYDRATE

This group of foods should be the main source of energy and form the basis of any meal.

Boosting meals with extra portions of starchy carbohydrates and vegetables can help to ensure a healthy balance with not too much energy from fat.

Wheat is a major source of starchy carbohydrate in this country. It is made into bread, biscuits, pasta, noodles, breakfast cereals, puddings and pastries as well as being used as an ingredient to thicken soups and sauces.

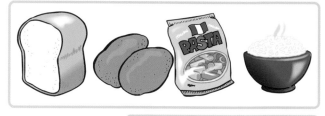

The best source of energy in the diet is starchy carbohydrates. Refined carbohydrates are those from more refined products such as white flour. Unrefined carbohydrates are less highly processed such as wholemeal flour for use in making wholemeal bread.

To ensure that about 50% of the energy for a meal is provided from carbohydrate, it is important to use extra carbohydrates:

- ♦ rice of all types can be served as part of a dish such as a risotto or accompanying a dish. Rice salads can be offered. It can also form the basis of puddings;
- ♦ potatoes can be served as part of a dish such as shepherd's pie, curries, salads or as accompaniments.
- ♦ bread of various types can be offered as an accompaniment. Paratha, ciabbatas and croissants are all high in fat;

Need to encourage diet high in starchy carbohydrates

- • **Bread**
- • **Potatoes**
- • **Pasta**
- • **Rice**
- • **Cereals**

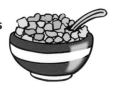

Plenty of fruit & vegetables

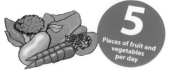

5 Pieces of fruit and vegetables per day

TERMS USED WITH CARBOHYDRATE FOODS

- Starchy carbohydrates
- Sugary carbohydrates or sugars
- Refined carbohydrates
- Unrefined carbohydrates

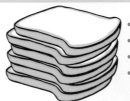

- Sugars
- Intrinsic sugar
- Extrinsic sugar
- Non-milk extrinsic sugar

♦ noodles can form a basis of stir-fries made with a minimum amount of fat;

♦ pasta can be served as an accompaniment such as spaghetti with Bolognese, or as macaroni bakes or even as milk puddings;

♦ couscous can be used in wraps, as salads and with stews;

♦ oats can be used to thicken dishes like casseroles. A handful of oats can be added to crumbles and biscuits to give an extra crunch to the dish; and

♦ snacks of popcorn, plain biscuits, rice cakes, currant buns, breadsticks and cornchips are all good sources of starchy carbohydrate.

CARBOHYDRATES

Refined carbohydrates
- **processed e.g. white flour**

Unrefined carbohydrates
- **less highly processed e.g. wholemeal bread**

Sugars have been implicated in causing dental decay. Intrinsic sugars are those which are found as part of the structure of a food such as sugars found in fruits.

MEAT, FISH AND ALTERNATIVES

This group of foods is considered to be one of the main sources of protein.

In order to limit the amount of fat from this group of foods, lean meat should be used rather than fatty ones. It is recommended to include fish three times a week if possible.

Red meat

The amount of fat in red meat has been considerably reduced over the last few decades in the UK, with the fat content of the carcase being reduced by over 30% for pork, 15% for beef and by 10% for lamb from the 1950s to the 1990s.

These reductions in fat for red meat have been achieved by breeding techniques on the farm selecting for leaner animals. New butchery techniques, which trim off most of the fat, have also contributed to the reduction in the fat content of red meat.

Fully trimmed raw beef typically contains only 5% fat, fully trimmed raw pork only 4% fat and fully trimmed raw lamb only 8% fat.

For example, 100g of beef, average trimmed lean raw, contains 5.1g of fat, 100g of pork, average trimmed lean raw, contains 4.0g of fat and 100g of lamb, average trimmed raw, contains 8.3g of fat. Many of the packs of meat found are much lower than this with joints of fully trimmed pork containing less than 2% fat.

Therefore lean red meat can be easily included in even the lowest fat diets.

About half of the fat found in red meat is in the unsaturated form, which is believed to be healthier. Surveys show that meat is a major contributor of monounsaturated fat in the diet. Monounsaturated fats are the type found in olive oil. Useful amounts of polyunsaturated fatty acids are found in red meat. Polyunsaturated fat is associated with a lower risk of heart disease.

Attention has focused on the omega-3 fatty acids as evidence suggests they are beneficial in conditions such as rheumatoid arthritis. While these fatty acids are particularly abundant in oily fish, however, meat also provides them. In Britain we get approximately 20% of our intake from meat.

Lean red meat is an excellent source of protein. Cooked lean red meat contains approximately 30% protein. Thus meat provides a significant contribution to our protein needs.

Protein is required for growth and repair of body tissues. During pregnancy and the first four months of breastfeeding extra protein is recommended. Anyone who has suffered an injury or undergone an operation may need extra protein. Extra protein is also recommended for sportsmen and sportswomen.

Red meat provides a valuable contribution to the amount of iron in the diet. Iron is an essential nutrient. It acts as an oxygen carrier in the blood and muscle. A lack of dietary iron can contribute to iron deficiency anaemia.

There are two forms of dietary iron: haem-iron and non-haem iron. The iron in red meat is in the haem form, and is well absorbed while the iron in cereals, vegetables and fruit are poorly absorbed. However if meat is eaten at the same meal as other foods then it actually enhances the absorption of iron from these other foods. It is important that those who do not take meat ensure they take adequate iron from other sources.

Zinc is a vital component in the functioning of the immune system of the body, which helps to fight diseases and infections. Men need more zinc than women.

The most reliable source of zinc in the diet is from meat. Zinc in meat is in a form which is easily absorbed.

Red meat is a good source of selenium, which has been recognised to be an important antioxidant. It is considered to be important in protecting against coronary heart disease and cancers.

Meat is an important source of B vitamins. Pork is a particularly rich source of thiamin.

Red meat is a major source of vitamin B_{12}. This vitamin is only found in foods of animal origin. Those who do not take red meat need to ensure they take enough of this important vitamin from another source.

Lean red meat has been shown to be a valuable source of vitamin D. Most people obtain adequate amounts of vitamin D by the action of sunlight on the skin. But for those who do not go out of doors such as those who live in residential homes or who wear clothes that fully conceal them, a source of vitamin D such as that found in lean red meat is needed. Other groups who are vulnerable to inadequate levels of vitamin D can be those who do not eat meat or oily fish.

Fish

Fish is a good source of protein and iron. Oily fish is a good source of omega-3 fatty acids. Additionally oily fish is a useful source of vitamins A and D. This can be especially useful for elderly

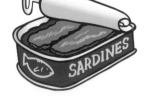

people as cans of fish are a useful store-cupboard stand-by.

Canned fish with bones such as sardines and salmon also provides calcium.

White fish such as cod and plaice is low in fat but still provides protein and some iron.

The normal portion guide for fish is 2-4oz (50-100g) of oily fish and 4-6oz oz (100g-150g) of white fish.

Unfortunately much of the white fish is sold in a convenient form with batter and breadcrumb coatings or with a sauce, all of which provide extra fat in the diet.

Eggs

Eggs are a good source of protein and are easy and convenient to prepare.

Those with raised cholesterol levels may also be advised to restrict the amount of foods containing cholesterol. The main sources of cholesterol are egg yolks, liver and shell fish.

Peas, beans and lentils and nuts

Peas, beans and lentils are regarded as pulses and a good source of protein in the diet. They are especially important in the diet of vegetarians and vegans.

The iron contained in pulses is in the non-haem form and is thus poorly absorbed. Vitamin C assists the absorption of this type of iron while high-fibre foods such as wheat bran can inhibit it.

Pulses also contain soluble fibre which is the type of fibre that can have beneficial effect on lowering blood cholesterol levels.

Nuts also provide protein and are a good source of polyunsaturated and monounsaturated fatty acids.

MILK AND DAIRY FOODS

This group is a major source of calcium and protein in the diet. As it is important to try and reduce the fat content of the diet in respect of milk and dairy foods the following is helpful:

♦ use skimmed or semi-skimmed milk, up to one pint a day;
♦ use cottage cheese. Avoid hard and cream cheeses. A sprinkle of Parmesan cheese can give the flavour to sauces etc. without excessive amounts of fat; and
♦ sauces can be made using cornflour to thicken them rather than a roux.

FOODS CONTAINING FATS AND FOODS CONTAINING SUGAR

The preferred source of energy for health is carbohydrates and around 50% of our energy should be taken from these. This leaves 15% of the energy to be obtained from protein foods.

It is recommended that we do not eat too much saturated fat because of links with heart disease. For the average adult in the UK, it is considered that women should not take more than about 70g of fat per day and men about 90g.

There has been an increased demand from the consumer in Britain for foods which are lower in fat. Examples of numerous low fat products are seen on the supermarket shelf.

Question to determine progress

Describe malnutrition and give examples found in the United Kingdom. **See answer in the appendix.**

9 Therapeutic diets

Some people who have various medical conditions require a 'therapeutic', 'special' or 'modified diet'. Such diets are usually prescribed by the person's general practitioner or consultant and the diet is usually advised by a State Registered Dietitian who will provide information based on medical information from the doctor and knowledge of food and nutrition.

The dietitian will usually advise on the type of foods to be included and avoided as part of the diet. Cooking methods, meal times, snacks and menus will usually be discussed. Items such as food labels and how to examine these as well as suitable brands of food are also usually covered. Some patients may require to be given a prescription for specialised dietary products such as gluten-free bread. Such special dietary products are usually prescribed to people by their GP in much the same way as medicines are prescribed.

The proportions of the different food groups as found in the 'Balance of Good Health' may not be appropriate for those on a special therapeutic diet. For example, those requiring a high calorie diet may be encouraged to take more of foods containing fat and those containing sugar.

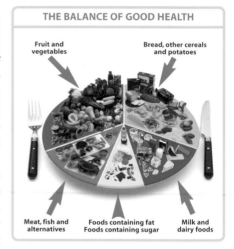

THE BALANCE OF GOOD HEALTH

Fruit and vegetables

Bread, other cereals and potatoes

Meat, fish and alternatives

Foods containing fat
Foods containing sugar

Milk and dairy foods

DIETS FOR PEOPLE WITH DIABETES

Diabetes mellitus is a medical condition which affects a large number of people. Insulin is normally produced by the pancreas and this assists the body to utilise the sugars (mainly glucose) derived from carbohydrate foods. There are two main types of diabetes mellitus:

♦ **Type 1** This used to be called 'juvenile' or 'insulin dependent' and usually occurs in younger people under 30 years of age.

♦ **Type 2** This used to be called 'maturity onset' or 'non-insulin dependent diabetes' and usually occurs in older people, especially in those who are overweight.

In those with diabetes mellitus the insulin that is produced is in too small quantities (such as occurs in Type 1 diabetes) or in a form that does not work correctly (as occurs in Type 2 diabetes). Therefore sugar (glucose), derived from the carbohydrate foods that are eaten, is not able to be used, builds up in the blood and eventually spills over into the urine.

Those with Type 1 diabetes mellitus require insulin and a diet for their control while those with Type 2 diabetes usually only require a diet, or a diet and tablets, for its control.

Aims of diet are to:

♦ control the level of sugar (glucose) in the blood;

♦ maintain the body weight within normal levels;

♦   maintain good nutrition and prevent complications; and
♦   to enable growth to occur in children.

Principles of diet:
♦   avoid added sugar in teas and coffees, on cereals and in sweets and chocolate;
♦   choose low sugar or sugar-reduced products such as soft drinks, jellies, 'whippy' style puddings, custards and jams;
♦   reduce the fat content of the diet by choosing lean cuts of meat and preparing these without extra fat. Provide alternatives to fried foods such as oven-baked rather than deep-fat fried chips, use grilled rather than fried bacon, avoid pastry dishes; use low-fat spreads in making sponges and scones;
♦   provide five portions of fruit and vegetables per day. Choose fresh fruit or fruit canned in fruit juices. Include puddings based on fruit such as fruit salads, crumbles made with low fat spread, less sugar and added oats, fruit cobblers made with low fat spreads and a mixture of white and wholemeal flour, pies with a thin 'low fat' pastry lid;
♦   provide plenty of starchy carbohydrate e.g. bread, potatoes, rice, pasta;
♦   provide regular meals; and
♦   diabetic foods are not recommended.

DIETS FOR PEOPLE REQUIRING A LOW FAT DIET

Individuals may require a low fat diet for various reasons.
1.   Many people who have raised cholesterol levels require a diet low in saturated fat to help reduce these levels. Those who have raised cholesterol levels are thought to be at an increased risk of heart disease.
2.   People who are suffering from gall bladder disease or gall stones may find their symptoms are eased by the use of a low fat diet.
3.   Those with disorders of the pancreas or liver may be advised to keep to a low fat diet to assist in controlling their symptoms.
4.   Some people with digestive disorders do not easily tolerate fat.
5.   People with diabetes and also those who are overweight are advised to take diets low in fat.

There are different types of fat found in the diet (saturated fats, polyunsaturated fats and monounsaturated fats), but the main aim of a low fat diet is to reduce all types of fat.

Aims of a low fat diet are to:
♦   reduce the fat level of the diet to a maximum of 40-50g per day for adults. However some people may be recommended a lower amount by their dietitian or doctor;
♦   maintain the body weight within normal levels: as fat is a concentrated source of energy, unless plenty of starchy carbohydrate foods such as bread, potatoes, pasta or rice are given an excessive amount of weight may be lost; and
♦   maintain good nutrition.

Principles of diet:
♦   use lean meat such as fully trimmed beef, pork and lamb. Avoid oily fish such as sardines or pilchards and use white fish such as cod, plaice or coley. Eggs have fat in

the yolk so their use should be restricted to no more than three per week. Nuts are rich in fat and should be avoided;

♦ provide food that is low in fat by avoiding foods such as fried foods, pastries, cream, deep fried foods and roast potatoes;

♦ substitute thick-cut oven chips and dry roast potatoes, made by brushing potatoes with a little oil and then cooking as usual, for those cooked in the normal way with fat;

♦ avoid pastry dishes and cakes. Instead provide meringues, fruit charlottes, low fat sponges, currant buns and crumbles made with low fat spread;

♦ use skimmed or semi-skimmed milk in drinks and on cereals and also for making 'whippy' type puddings, rice pudding and custards;

♦ ensure that foods contain adequate calories by providing large portions of rice, bread, potatoes and pasta as well as plain biscuits; and

♦ apart from olives and avocado, fruit and vegetables contain no fat.

Those with raised cholesterol levels may also be advised to restrict the amount of foods containing cholesterol. The main sources of cholesterol are egg yolks, liver and shellfish.

DIETS FOR PEOPLE REQUIRING A LOW FAT DIET

- Individuals may require a low fat diet for various reasons
  - **People who have raised cholesterol levels**
  - **People who are suffering from gall bladder disease**
  - **Those with disorders of the pancreas or liver**
  - **Some people with digestive disorders do not easily tolerate fat**
  - **People with diabetes and also those who are overweight**

- Aims of diet
  - **To reduce the fat level of the diet to a maximum of 40-50g per day for adults**
  - **Provide plenty of starchy carbohydrate foods**

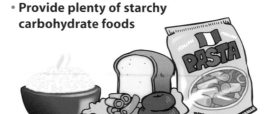

DIET FOR RAISED LIPIDS *(CHOLESTEROL)*

- Avoid
  - **Excessive amounts of saturated fat in the diet, for example:**
    - **Full fat cheese, cream cheese, pastry, pork pies, sausage rolls, cream, full cream, milk, fried foods and fat on meat**

- If there are also raised triglycerides
  - **Avoid excess refined carbohydrates such as sugar and items containing them, for example:**
    - **Sweets, chocolate, cream biscuits, toffees, Danish pastries and cakes**

Boosting meals with extra portions of starchy carbohydrates and vegetables can help to ensure a healthy balance with not too much energy from fat.

FOOD INTOLERANCES

The whole area of food allergies and food intolerances is a complex and controversial one. There are many medical problems which are related to food intolerances.

Coeliac disease is the most common form of gluten intolerance but there are other conditions which benefit from a wheat- or gluten-free diet.

FOOD ALLERGIES AND INTOLERANCES

- **Adverse reaction to food, beverage, ingredient or additive in a food**
- **Occurs every time that the food is taken**
- **Includes food allergies and digestive enzyme defects, pharmacological reactions and other non-specific reactions to foods**

- **20% of the population considered they react adversely**
- **Only about 5-8% of children and 1-2% of adults are affected**

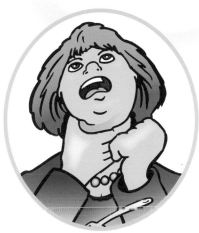

FOOD ALLERGIES & INTOLERANCES

- Disorders which can be due to intolerances
  - **Asthma and wheezing**
  - **Rhinitis with a continually runny nose**
  - **Eczema**
  - **Autism**
  - **Coeliac disease & dermatitis herpetiformis**
  - **Diarrhoea**
  - **Cystitis**
  - **Anaphylactic shock**
  - **Irritable Bowel Syndrome (IBS)**
  - **Hyperactivity or ADHD**
  - **Constipation**
  - **Depression and irritability**
  - **Migraines and headaches**
  - **Rheumatoid arthritis**
  - **Skin rashes**

Definitions

Food intolerance is a condition whereby a person is adversely affected by a food, beverage, ingredient or additive in a food. This adverse reaction occurs every time that the food is taken even if the food is disguised in a meal. The term food intolerance includes food allergies, digestive enzyme defects, pharmacological reactions and other non-specific reactions to foods.

Disorders which can be due to food intolerances

There are a number of disorders which have been considered to be due to food intolerances, and these include a whole range of conditions.

Food causing intolerance

All types of foods and ingredients can cause reactions depending on the individual.

Wheat and gluten intolerances

The most important intolerance to gluten is that of coeliac disease whereby a reaction occurs in the mucosal lining of the small intestine. As a result the villi become flattened and hence have a reduced capacity for absorption. A small percentage of people with coeliac disease require a wheat-free diet rather than just a gluten-free diet. Dermatitis herpetiformis is a skin condition where itchy blisters form and treatment is by a gluten-free diet. For both conditions gluten-free products are available on prescription.

Gluten is found in products containing wheat. Some individuals such as those with coeliac disease have an intolerance to gluten. Coeliac disease can result in unpleasant gastrointestinal symptoms and the only treatment is a gluten-free diet. For people requiring such a diet, gluten-free products are available from their doctor on prescription.

Aims of a wheat- and gluten-free diet are to:
♦ prevent any symptoms caused by the intolerance to gluten;
♦ maintain the body weight within normal levels;
♦ maintain good nutrition;
♦ prevent complications; and
♦ in children, enable growth to occur.

Principles of diet:
♦ gluten is found in all wheat products and also rye. Therefore any foods made from these need to be excluded;
♦ bread needs to be replaced by a gluten-free bread;
♦ biscuits should be replaced by gluten-free ones;
♦ gluten-free pasta should be used instead of ordinary pasta;
♦ gluten-free flour, or cornflour, should be used in the place of ordinary flour for baking and thickening sauces; and
♦ meat, fish, eggs, cheese, fruit, vegetables, rice, milk and potatoes can all be used as part of a gluten-free diet.

Some people with other conditions such as IBS or rheumatoid arthritis may also have an intolerance to wheat. Although a wheat-free diet can eliminate symptoms, the wheat-free products are not available on prescription.

Some people who have an intolerance to wheat may also have an intolerance to another food such as milk.

Food causing intolerance

- **Peanuts** *(& items containing them)*
- **Tree nuts** *(e.g. almonds, walnuts & brazils)*
- **Shellfish** *(e.g. prawns)*
- **Eggs** *(& foods containing them)*
- **Lactose** *(from milk and milk products)*
- **Gluten** *(from wheat, rye & barley)*
- **Wheat** *(& items containing it)*
- **Citrus fruit and juices**
- **Sesame** *(including oils & seeds)*
- **Sunflower** *(seeds and oils)*
- **Poppy seeds found in bread and biscuits**
- **Molluscs** *(snails and cockles)*
- **Beans** *(soya beans and soya milk)*
- **Peas and lentils**

GLUTEN-FREE DIETS

- **Coeliac disease and dermatitis herpetiformis**
  - **Gluten-free or wheat-free products such as breads, biscuits, flours and pasta can be prescribed for those with medically diagnosed coeliac disease or dermatitis herpetiformis**

- **Other conditions**
  - **Schizophrenia**
  - **Multiple sclerosis**
  - **Depression**
  - **Skin conditions**
  - **Bowel problems, e.g. IBS**
  - **Autism or Crohn's disease**

DIETS FOR PEOPLE WITH DEMENTIA

The number of people with dementia is expected to rise, which will increase the demand that they place both on community and residential care.

Dementia can affect coordination and thus the ability to use cutlery and to peel or unwrap food, as well as an inability to sit for long periods. This can mean that sufferers need to be able to eat while moving around.

They can lose their appetite as well as being easily distracted from eating and losing their interest in foods. This means that people may forget that they have just eaten and demand another meal or insist that they have eaten when they have not.

These effects can cause a diminished intake and thus insufficient calories, protein, vitamins, minerals and fluid.

Aims of a diet for people with dementia are to:
♦   enable sufficient nutrition to be taken in an easily eaten form;
♦   maintain the body weight within normal levels;
♦   provide adequate fluid; and
♦   maintain good nutrition.

Principles of diet:
♦   provide food that is easy to eat;
♦   ensure that foods contain adequate calories;
♦   provide foods that are easy to eat from the hand; and
♦   give reminders about eating.

DIETS WHICH ARE HIGH IN IRON

A lack of iron in the diet can contribute to iron deficiency anaemia. This can cause symptoms of tiredness and listlessness. It can also delay wound healing.

Women of child-bearing age and elderly people are particularly susceptible to iron deficiency anaemia.

Aims of a diet high in iron are to:
♦   provide adequate quantities of iron in the diet;
♦   maintain good nutrition; and
♦   prevent complications.

Principles of diet:
♦   provide a good source of iron in the diet. The iron in red meat (beef, pork and lamb) is in the haem form, which is easily absorbed. Offal such as liver and kidney contains even greater quantities of haem iron. Another advantage of red meat is that when it is eaten at the same time as other foods it actually enhances the absorption of iron from those foods. Fish also contains some iron in the haem form;
♦   pulses such as peas, dried beans and lentils, eggs, nuts and fish all contain some iron. The iron is in a non-haem form which is less well absorbed. For those who do not eat meat it is important that they take adequate amounts of these foods to provide sufficient dietary iron;

◆ vitamin C helps to enhance the absorption of iron so provide plenty (five portions) of fruit and vegetables per day. Give fruit juice with meals to boost iron absorption; and

◆ although liver is a rich source of iron, due to its also being a rich source of vitamin A, it is not suitable for those who are pregnant as high levels of vitamin A in pregnancy are harmful to the foetus.

DIETS WHICH ARE HIGH IN CALCIUM

A lack of calcium in the diet can contribute to conditions such as osteoporosis. This can cause a fragility of the bones, which makes them more susceptible to fractures. The group which is most susceptible is women past the age of 50 years and also older men.

Osteoporosis is a complicated disorder but a lack of calcium as well as low levels of female sex hormones (such as occur after the menopause), a sedentary lifestyle with little exercise, smoking, being underweight and certain medications such as the long-term use of steroids are all factors which contribute.

Calcium is found in milk, cheese and yoghurts and foods containing them. Fish with small bones such as pilchards and sardines, white bread and dried fruit also contain some calcium.

Vitamin D is needed for the body to absorb calcium. Most people obtain enough vitamin D from the action of sunlight on their skin. However those who do not go out of doors need to ensure a dietary source of vitamin D. Butter, spreads, red meat and offal, full cream milk, eggs and oily fish all contain vitamin D.

Aims of a diet high in calcium are to:
◆ provide plenty of calcium;
◆ maintain good nutrition; and
◆ ensure that, for those who do not go out of doors, the diet contains enough vitamin D.

Principles of diet:
◆ provide at least a pint of milk per day. Skimmed and semi-skimmed milks contain similar quantities of calcium to that of full cream milk;
◆ however, full cream milk contains vitamin D as well. Use the milk in drinks, on cereals, in soups, sauces, and puddings;
◆ extra calcium can be added to milk itself, soups, sauces and puddings by adding a spoonful of dried milk powder. Mix well to thoroughly disperse powder;
◆ include cheese as sandwich fillings, on vegetables and as snacks;
◆ provide a portion of meat or fish or eggs daily; and
◆ for those who do not take dairy products, ensure that calcium enriched soya milks are included.

DIETS FOR THOSE WHO ARE HIV POSITIVE

People who are HIV positive have an immune system that is not functioning correctly and therefore they are susceptible to all sorts of infections.

Additionally weight loss can occur which can be due to an altered metabolic rate, malabsorption and decreased intake of food.

Due to the malabsorption, gastrointestinal problems such as diarrhoea can occur.

Principles of diet:

- provide food that is freshly and hygienically prepared;
- avoid such foods as raw or undercooked meat and fish, undercooked or raw eggs or foods containing them such as mousses and unpasteurised milk and cheeses;
- ensure that water is from a safe source and that for those requiring it boiled water is used for all drinks, cooking and washing of foods;
- provide foods that are tempting and adequate in all nutrients;
- give regular snacks so that the diet is high in calories; and
- use any supplements and calorie sources in meals that are provided by the doctor.

DIETS FOR PEOPLE WHO ARE HIV POSITIVE

- Their immune system is not functioning correctly
- Susceptible to all sorts of infections
- Additionally, weight loss can occur which can be due to an altered metabolic rate, malabsorption and decreased intake of food
- Due to the malabsorption gastrointestinal problems such as diarrhoea can occur

- Principles of diet
  - Provide food that is freshly and hygienically prepared
  - Avoid such foods as raw or undercooked meat and fish, undercooked or raw eggs or foods containing them
  - Give regular snacks so that the diet is high in calories

HIGH CALORIE DIETS

High calorie diets are those which are also high in energy. A high calorie diet is needed for those who are underweight. Such people may have lost weight over a long period of time, because of illness or even a lack of appetite. Those who have had an operation or serious illness will often need a high calorie diet to promote healing to occur. Those who are hyperactive and always on the move will also need a to have a high calorie diet.

To encourage a high calorie intake, tempting high calorie meals with extra snacks between meals are needed.

Often the doctor on the advice of a dietitian may prescribe various supplements. These can often be used in cooking.

Aims of a diet high in calories are to:

- provide a diet high in calories;
- maintain good nutrition;
- promote weight gain and prevent weight loss; and
- make full use of any prescribed supplements.

Principles of diet:

- provide tempting and appetising meals. These include casseroles, curries, and roast meals with Yorkshire puddings, lasagnes and pies;
- provide vegetables supplemented with a pat of butter;

- ◆ use sauces such as white sauce made with full cream milk and extra cream;
- ◆ add milk powder to milk, soups, sauces and custards to boost the calorie intake;
- ◆ boost sandwich fillings with extras such as grated cheese and mayonnaise to ham sandwiches;
- ◆ give cream, custards and ice creams with desserts; and
- ◆ provide cakes, scones, crisps and chocolate as snacks.

PURÉED DIETS

People who have a swallowing difficulty or have had dental treatment may need their food to be puréed or liquidised.

Aims of puréed diets are to:
- ◆ enable sufficient nutrition to be taken in a puréed form;
- ◆ maintain the body weight within normal levels;
- ◆ provide adequate fluid by giving thickened liquids if required; and
- ◆ maintain good nutrition.

Principles of diet:
- ◆ provide food that is smooth; and
- ◆ ensure that foods contain adequate calories.

DIETS WHICH ARE HIGH IN FIBRE

A lack of fibre non-starch polysaccharide, roughage or residue as it is called) can lead to bowel problems such as constipation and diverticular disease. To prevent constipation and avoid the symptoms of diverticular disease it is important to take a diet high in fibre. Also plenty of fluid (approximately two litres (three pints per day) is important.

There are two types of dietary fibre:
- ◆ soluble fibre, found in oats, lentils, peas, dried beans, fruit, vegetables, barley and rye; and
- ◆ insoluble fibre, found in wholemeal bread, brown pasta, bran-based cereals, rice and corn.

Adequate amounts of fibre are also important aspects of diets for people with diabetes and raised cholesterol levels. Anyone who is overweight will also find a high-fibre diet of benefit, as it is more filling.

Aims of high-fibre diets are to:
- ◆ provide plenty of fibre;
- ◆ provide plenty of fluid;
- ◆ alleviate symptoms; and
- ◆ maintain good nutrition.

Principles of diet:
- ◆ provide at least a two litres of fluid (three pints) per day. Try to provide a variety of

fluids. Water is especially important;
♦ ensure that five portions of fruit and vegetables excluding potatoes (about 500g or 1lb) per day are provided;
♦ offer wholemeal bread and high-fibre white breads as alternatives;
♦ offer porridge and high-fibre, wholewheat, cereals at breakfast times;
♦ offer dried fruit as snacks. Also offer cereal bars, bran, oat and digestive biscuits and fruit cakes between meals; and
♦ try to add extra lentils, dried peas or oats to casseroles and stews to thicken them and provide extra fibre. Even an extra can of baked beans will boost the amount of soluble fibre in a dish.

Resources on special diets

Local dietitians will be able to provide further information on therapeutic special diets. They will also be able to provide ways of using supplements in cooking dishes.

DIETS WHICH ARE LOW IN RESIDUE

Some people who have gastrointestinal problems require a low residue diet. This diet is also low in fibre.

Such diets are usually only used for a short time while someone recovers from something such as surgery on the digestive tract.

There are two types of dietary fibre:
♦ soluble fibre, which is found in oats, lentils, peas, dried beans, fruit and vegetables;
♦ insoluble fibre, which is found in wholemeal bread, brown pasta and bran based cereals.

The soluble type of fibre is soft and unlikely to irritate the digestive tract and therefore can usually be included.

It is also important that fruit is peeled and items with lots of seeds avoided. Hard pieces of food such as found in granary bread may also upset. Nuts and seeds should be avoided. Hard pieces of chips and roast potato are also likely to upset, as will highly spiced food.

Aims of low residue diets are to:
♦ avoid foods with insoluble fibre, for example, wholemeal bread, brown rice, brown pasta, wholegrain cereals, such as bran flakes and muesli;
♦ provide plenty of fluid;
♦ alleviate symptoms; and
♦ maintain good nutrition.

Principles of diet:
♦ provide white bread and rolls and lower-fibre breakfast cereals such as cornflakes and Rice Krispies;
♦ ensure that plenty of potatoes cooked without fat, rice and white pasta are provided;
♦ peel vegetables before cooking;
♦ give cooked fruit dishes such as apple charlottes, fruit canned in syrup, stewed fruit and peeled fresh fruit; and
♦ provide puddings such as sponges and milk puddings rather than heavy fruit cakes.

MAOI DIETS

MAOI drugs (Mono Amine Oxidase Inhibitors) are often given to people for depression. Certain foods contain amines and these can interact with the MAOI drugs in a dangerous way. Therefore foods containing amines must be carefully excluded from the diet. Amines are found in cheese (especially strong cheeses such as mature cheddar and stilton), game which has been hung such as rabbits, grouse and pheasant, meat and yeast extracts (such as Oxo, Bovril, Marmite, stock cubes and sauce mixes), pickled herrings, textured vegetable protein (TVP) and alcohol.

Aims of MAOI diets are to:
- carefully exclude all foods containing amines;
- provide a good and varied diet; and
- maintain good nutrition.

Principles of diet:
- check labels for sources of amines such as yeast extracts;
- use herbs, spices, meat juices, home-made stock, and well cooked onion to flavour gravies, soups, casseroles and stews;
- use a variety of sandwich fillings including salads, cold meats (for example, lamb and mint), ham, chicken, turkey, salmon, sardines, pilchards, tuna and peanut butter. Try making wraps and filling with something such as shredded pork and beef. For other easily eaten snacks include pizzas, quiches, sausage rolls etc.;
- use fresh meats rather than game or dishes containing game;
- provide sparkling drinks instead of alcohol; and
- avoid alcohol in cooking.

Resources

Local dietitians can provide advice on diet, cooking methods and suitable foods.

Pharmacists can also produce a list of foods that react with the MAOI medication as well as lists of specially prescribable foods.

Question to determine progress

Describe the main principles of a diet for someone with type 2 diabetes who is overweight. **See answer in the appendix.**

MAOI DIETS

- **MAOI drugs (Mono Amine Oxidase Inhibitors) are often given to people for depression**

- **Certain foods contain amines and these can interact**

- **Amines are found in:**
  - **cheese – especially strong cheeses**
  - **game – such as rabbit, grouse and pheasant**
  - **meat and yeast extracts - such as stock cubes**
  - **pickled herrings**
  - **textured vegetable protein**
  - **alcohol**

10 Ethnic minority groups and their dietary requirements

Britain is a multicultural country with many different nationalities represented. These cultural groups often have their own dietary patterns.

People may also follow a particular diet for ethical reasons, for example, those who do not believe that animals should be used for food may follow a vegan diet.

With increasing travel, food and catering in the UK have taken on an international flavour. This is often of great appeal to many cultural groups. For example, someone who is a Hindu, and a strict lacto-vegetarian, may enjoy a pizza or Chinese stir-fry dish.

Even if someone says he or she is a vegetarian, it is helpful to establish what this means. Sometimes people who say they are vegetarians will happily eat beefburgers or dishes containing minced meat but who find joints of meat and hence slices of meat or chops totally unacceptable. Therefore it is always important to ensure that the diet is fully discussed and no assumptions made.

The principal minority cultural and ethical groups are:

◆ Muslims;	◆ Hindus;
◆ Afro-Caribbean;	◆ West African;
◆ Chinese;	◆ Vietnamese;
◆ Jewish;	◆ Vegetarians and vegans.

Numbers from different cultural groups

The breakdown of the figures regarding cultural groups from the 1991 census showed that over 3,000,000 people were of a minority ethnic origin.

The largest group is of South Asian origin, followed by those of African-Caribbean origin.

However the concentration of different ethnic groups varies considerably throughout the UK with concentrations in some parts of London and cities such as Bradford. Also within a town or city there may be certain areas where schools have large numbers of pupils from different cultural groups while another school may have few.

DIFFERENT CULTURAL GROUPS

South Asian people

South Asians originate from the Indian subcontinent. The three main religions of South Asians are:

◆ Hinduism;
◆ Islam; and
◆ Sikhism.

Hindus rarely eat beef and many will not eat other meat or fish. Some less strict Hindus will eat lamb, kid, poultry or white fish. Very strict Hindus will not take any eggs or any foods containing meat products such as gelatine. They may be very concerned to know what is in a dish and need reassurance that everything is of vegetable origin.

Muslims follow the religion of Islam. They do not take any food or products from the pig. Shellfish or fish without fins or scales are also not acceptable.

Sikhs may be less strict than Muslims or Hindus. They tend to be lacto-vegetarians but some will take lamb, kid, poultry and fish. Most Sikhs do not take beef or pork.

The diet of many young people from South Asia may focus more on a lacto-vegetarian diet due to concerns regarding the type and origins of meat. Meat is a major source of readily absorbed iron in the diet, which is essential to the body. Lacto-vegetarian diets can be well-balanced provided that an adequate source of iron is included as pulses, lentils and legumes.

Vitamin B_{12} is derived from foods of animal origin such as milk, meat and eggs. Therefore if no meat or eggs are taken in the diet, it is important to include a source of vitamin B_{12} such as that from dairy products.

Vitamin D is required by the body to enable calcium absorption to occur. Most people derive vitamin D by the action of sunlight on the skin. Vitamin D is also derived from meat and fish. For those who wear clothing that covers the body and who do not take meat or fish alternative sources of vitamin D such as full fat milk, supplemented spreads or margarines should be included.

African-Caribbean people

The diet of the African-Caribbeans may vary considerably between individuals, but in general there are few dietary restrictions. There are two main religious groups:

♦ Seventh-Day Adventists; and
♦ Rastafarians.

Both groups are usually vegetarian, but Rastafarians may take fish and shun foods which are processed.

A varied vegetarian diet can be provided to young people from African–Caribbean cultural groups.

Hypertension (high-blood pressure) can be a problem found in adults from African–Caribbean origins. As excessive amounts of salt have been linked with this condition it is recommended that excess salt is not used in cooking nor salty foods provided.

Jewish people

Jewish people have a number of dietary restrictions and like Muslims do not take pork or shellfish. Animals must be slaughtered according to a 'Kosher' method (this type of meat is acceptable to some Muslims). Meat should not be cooked with milk, and meat and milk should not be consumed at the same meal.

Separate utensils and indeed separate kitchens are used for the preparation of meat and milk dishes in orthodox establishments.

Chinese and Vietnamese people

The diet of the population of China varies considerably. In general rice and noodles comprise the starchy component of the diet. Soya beans are used in a variety of ways, as are fruit and vegetables. Meat and fish are consumed but milk and milk products such as cheese are rarely taken. Indeed some people from Chinese backgrounds may not tolerate milk.

Therefore calcium from other sources such as supplemented soya milks and fish with small bones should be provided.

Fasting

Many of the religious groups observe various fasts. For example, Muslims fast from dawn to dusk during the period of Ramadan. While children are exempt from such fasts, they may elect to follow their religious tradition and fast, which can obviously cause problems at school with concentration lapses due to a lack of food.

Other groups such as followers of the Greek Orthodox faith may fast by not taking foods of animal origin in the period before Christmas and Easter. The period of Lent is a time when many give up something such as chocolate or other foods. Therefore menus need to be able to encompass these requirements with extra fruit instead of other types of desserts.

Diets for ethical reasons

Diets for ethical reasons are mainly those of vegetarians, vegans and also groups such as fruitarians.

Vegetarians

Approximately 3% of the population follow a vegetarian diet. Vegetarians normally eat no foods which necessitate the killing of animals, and thus they do not eat any meat or poultry or products containing them such as pastry made from lard or jelly made with gelatine. Some vegetarians eat fish while others do not.

The vegetarian group includes:

♦ Lacto-ovo-vegetarians who eat eggs and products containing eggs such as quiches, mousses, mayonnaises, omelettes, cakes and other baked goods made with eggs. They also take milk and items of food made from milk such as cheese, which is made using vegetarian rennet and yoghurts, fromage frais and ice cream.

♦ Lacto-vegetarians – those who take milk and milk products but no eggs.

♦ Demi-vegetarians – those who eat fish and some poultry such as chicken and turkey but no red meat.

> ### VEGANS/VEGETARIANS
>
> **VEGANS**
> - **avoid all meat, fish, eggs, dairy products and anything derived from animals**
>
> **LACTO-OVO-VEGETARIANS**
> - **avoid all meat and fish but eat eggs and dairy products**
>
> **DEMI-VEGETARIANS**
> - **avoid red meat but eat poultry, fish, eggs and dairy products**

Due to the lack of red meat in the diet of vegetarians they can be susceptible to iron deficiency anaemia particularly in those with high needs such as menstruating women. It is therefore important that the diet is carefully balanced to include vegetarian sources of iron such as pulses (peas, beans and lentils) as well as nuts, dried fruit and fortified breakfast cereals. A source of vitamin C such as in vegetables, fruit or fruit juice taken with meals will enhance the absorption of non-haem iron from foods such as cereal, nuts or pulses.

Vegans

Vegans eat no food of animal origin and thus take no meat, poultry, eggs, milk or dairy products. They take a wide range of nuts, pulses, fruit, vegetables and cereals. Many also eat such items as seaweeds.

The diet of vegans can also be low in certain nutrients. These include:

- iron, so it is particularly important that they take adequate iron from foods such as fortified breakfast cereals, pulses, nuts and dried fruit. Again a food such as fruit juice, which contains vitamin C, will enhance the absorption of non-haem iron from vegetable sources;

- vitamin B_{12} is only found in foods of animal origin, so the diet of vegans may be low in this (as vitamin B_{12} is found in milk and eggs it is not usually deficient in a vegetarian diet). Vegans can obtain vitamin B_{12} from items such as yeast extracts and foods containing them;

- calcium – can be low in vegan diets and therefore it is important than any soya milks used are fortified with calcium. Other vegan sources of calcium are bread (including white bread, as calcium is added to the white flour used), nuts, seeds such as sesame seeds or tahini, pulses such as peas, beans, lentils, chickpeas, dried fruits or green vegetables;

- vitamin D levels may be low in those who are vegan and do not go out of doors or who do not expose their skin to sunlight. In this situation they are unable to make vitamin D by the action of sunlight on the skin. Dietary sources of vitamin D are oily fish, egg yolk, meat, cream, butter and full fat milk. Sources of vitamin D suitable for vegans are fortified milk-free spreads and margarines as well as fortified breakfast cereals;

- some vegans have difficulty in obtaining enough protein and energy from their diet, especially in times of a high requirement such as during lactation or illness. Extra protein can be provided in the diet by using extra soya products and by using extra desserts such as cookies, flap jacks and other snacks made with ingredients which are not derived from animals; and

- infants and toddlers following a vegan diet must have it carefully balanced to enable them to grow properly. A vegan diet can be very bulky and difficult for very young children to eat. Therefore special consideration should be made for these and specially fortified soya milks produced for infants used instead of the usual ones available in supermarkets.

VEGANS
• **Exclude any animal-derived ingredients added to manufactured food, such as emulsifiers derived from animal fats (e.g. lecithin) and firming agents (e.g. gelatin)**
• **Vegan diets must ensure that they provide sufficient protein, vitamins and minerals; risk of iron deficiency**
• **Avoidance of dairy products can increase the risk of low intakes of calcium, vitamin B_2 and vitamin B_{12}**

Question to determine progress

Describe the main principles of a diet for a Hindu. Plan a day's menu for Hindu family of mother, father, grandmother and toddler of 2 years. **See answer in the appendix.**

11 Promoting healthy eating

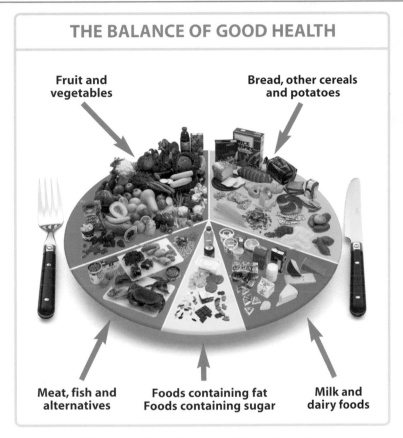

THE BALANCE OF GOOD HEALTH

Fruit and vegetables

Bread, other cereals and potatoes

Meat, fish and alternatives

Foods containing fat Foods containing sugar

Milk and dairy foods

The national food guide is called the 'Balance of Good Health'; it is a diagram of a plate model upon which there are segments representing the amounts of food, which would be found in a healthy balanced diet.

The segments include:

♦ fruit and vegetables;
♦ bread, other cereals and potatoes;
♦ meat, fish and alternatives;
♦ milk and dairy foods; and
♦ foods containing fat and foods containing sugar.

The plate model is promoted by the Food Standards Agency as the one to be used for nutritional education and promotion in Great Britain. Therefore one often sees the model displayed in health promotion clinics and dining rooms as well as numerous booklets on nutrition and health.

The 'Balance of Good Health' is fundamental to the concept of a healthy balanced diet. It shows that the diet should consist of plenty of fruit and vegetables; starchy carbohydrate foods such as bread, potatoes, pasta and rice; moderate portions of meat or fish or vegetarian alternatives such as pulses and nuts; and moderate amounts of dairy products such as skimmed milk and low fat yoghurts.

While for those who are ill, children or the elderly, the model may be adapted to give a greater proportion of calories and protein to assist recovery or promote growth and repair of the body, it does give a useful way of looking at the different food and nutrient groups.

Foods containing fat and foods containing sugar should be limited in the diet as these are the ones which can contribute to heath problems such as dental disease and coronary heart disease.

WAYS OF PROVIDING A HEALTHY DIET

Provide large portions of starchy carbohydrates

The preferred source of energy for health is carbohydrates and around 50% of our energy should be taken from these. Starchy carbohydrates have minimum amounts of fat in them and thus can be used to enhance the amount of energy derived from carbohydrate.

Fruit and vegetables group

One of the most important constituents of a healthy diet is fruit and vegetables.

The fruit and vegetables group includes all types of fruit and vegetables but excludes potatoes, which are considered to be a part of the group containing bread, other cereals and potatoes. Plantains or green bananas are also regarded as starchy carbohydrates and are therefore considered to be also part of the group containing potatoes.

Potatoes can be served as part of a dish as an accompaniment in various ways.

CARBOHYDRATES

Refined carbohydrates
*   **processed e.g. white flour**

Unrefined carbohydrates
*   **less highly processed e.g. wholemeal bread**

Vegetables such as pulses, i.e. dried or canned vegetables such as peas, beans and lentils, are considered to be a part of the meat, fish and alternative group. Pulses contain a good amount of protein and iron and thus can provide an alternative to meat in the diet of vegetarians and vegans.

Therefore it is important to ensure that menus provide adequate portions of both of these items. No matter what the age group, there should be plenty of fruit and vegetables included.

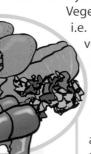

Fruit and vegetables
These provide vitamins
e.g. vitamin C, carotenes,
folates; some minerals
and dietary fibre

Research on nutrition and health has shown that a diet rich in fruit and vegetables can be beneficial in preventing the development of cancers and heart disease. This is felt not only to be due to vitamins like ascorbic acid (vitamin C) and beta-carotene (the precursor for vitamin A) but also because of other protective substances that fruit and vegetables contain.

It is quite easy for caterers to add extra vegetables to dishes. Not only are they nutritious but they are also relatively inexpensive. Vegetables can be added to curries, casseroles, in wraps, sandwiches, in stir-fries, as pizza toppings as well as accompaniments and in salads. Fruit can be added to breakfasts, snacks and puddings.

Fruit and vegetables are low in fat and again can help to adjust the contribution of energy from fat.

Protein foods

Normal portions of protein foods can be used. The protein foods include the section in the Balance of Good Health which includes meat, fish and alternatives and dairy foods. The meat, fish and alternatives are also major contributors of iron to the diet while the dairy foods are major contributors of calcium in the diet.

Milk and dairy foods are an important

Milk and dairy foods
* **These include milk, cheese, yoghurt, fromage frais**
* **They provide calcium, protein, vitamins A and D, vitamin B$_{12}$**

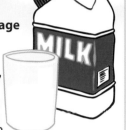

Meat, fish and alternatives
* **These include meat, poultry, fish, eggs, nuts, beans, pulses**
* **They provide iron, protein, B vitamins, especially B$_{12}$**

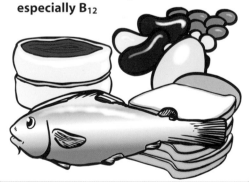

source of calcium, which is needed for the development of strong and healthy bones. It is during the teenage years that most of the calcium is deposited in the bones and thus this is a very important time for developing a strong skeleton. But a good source of calcium is required in the diet throughout life to maintain bone health.

It should be noted that skimmed milk is not suitable for children under five years of age as it does not contain enough calories. Full cream milk or semi-skimmed milk can be used for children below five years of age.

Some individuals are allergic or intolerant to cows' milk. This intolerance usually begins soon after birth. Most children grow out of this intolerance to cows' milk by the age of five years. Unfortunately for a few people this intolerance persists throughout life. Such children must not be given cows' milk. Soya milk or specially prescribed milks should be provided instead. Any soya milk used should be one of the ones supplemented with extra calcium.

The general principles of a healthy diet as regards protein foods are:
♦ use skimmed or semi-skimmed milk up to one pint a day;
♦ use cottage cheese. Avoid hard and cream cheeses. A sprinkle of Parmesan cheese can give the flavour to sauces etc without excessive amounts of fat;
♦ sauces can be made using cornflour to thicken them rather than roués;
♦ lean meat should be used rather than fatty ones; and
♦ include fish three times a week if possible.

Cooking methods which provide less fat are:

- steaming;
- braising;
- baking;
- grilling;
- barbecuing;
- poaching;
- casseroling;
- simmering;
- boiling;
- stewing; and
- dry frying without fat.

If frying is used for foods it is better to fry items such as plain cuts of meat as these will absorb less fat than any foods which have breadcrumb or batter coatings. Aim to have no more than 70-90g fat per day.

Also advocate low-fat spread rather than butter or full-fat margarine or spread. It is recommended that the percentage of the total amount of energy provided by fat in the diet is a maximum of 35%.

Fluid

The obvious fluid to take to replace body losses is water. It is vital to health that adequate amounts of fluids are provided.

Most adults require 1.5 to 2 litres (3 pints or 6-8 cups) of liquid per day. Fluids which contain large amounts of caffeine such as colas or coffee are not particularly hydrating. Alcohol is also not hydrating.

If sugary drinks such as colas are preferred to the low sugar varieties, it is best that these are taken at meal times to prevent the sugar encouraging tooth decay.

Meal Patterns

Regular meals are essential as part of a balanced diet. Such meals consist of breakfast, lunch and an evening meal. Meals can be either cooked or cold; both are equally nutritious.

BREAKFAST

Breakfast has long been recognised as a particularly important meal. The overnight fast from food, which occurs during sleep, is broken by eating breakfast and blood sugar levels are raised after eating breakfast. Breakfast is vital not from just a nutritional view but the way it enhances cognitive performance and hence the ability of children to learn. In some areas of the country, such as inner city areas, as few as 20% of children eat breakfast. Some schools already provide a form of breakfast with a morning break service of filled rolls and bacon sandwiches. Initiatives such as 'breakfast clubs' have been incorporated into more deprived areas. These are held prior to the start of the school day and provide a simple breakfast of cereals, toast and fruit juice for a small sum.

Breakfast is also a time when foods such as fibre-rich cereals and fruit juices can be taken.

Porridge can be a cheap and nutritious breakfast especially popular in winter time. Breakfast cereals chosen can be fortified with extra vitamins and minerals. Cereals can be served without sugar and sugar-free ones chosen.

Toast or bread with jam or marmalade is popular and low-fat spreads and low-sugar jams chosen for a more healthy option. Bagels, plain pancakes and croissants can also add variety. Croissants are relatively high in fat because of the butter they contain.

Obviously fried breakfasts can make a treat but can be a rich source of fat in the diet. Bacon and sausages can be grilled or oven baked instead of fried and served with fibre-rich items such as baked beans, tomatoes or mushrooms.

LUNCH

In the past this was frequently a cooked meal but while cooked meals may be popular if available at school or in the staff restaurant most people have insufficient time to cook at lunchtime.

Often snack meals such as sandwiches with a variety of fillings are eaten. The use of wholemeal bread will provide more fibre than white. Pitta breads and wraps can give added variety. Fillings can incorporate some salad vegetables. The use of low-fat mayonnaises and spreads helps to reduce the fat content of sandwiches.

Sandwiches can be accompanied by a side salad or fresh fruit or a dessert such as low-fat yoghurt, rather than potato crisps, chocolate or cakes every day.

Other quickly-prepared meals are soups, salads, jacket potatoes, slices of pizza or quiche served with a side salad.

EVENING MEAL

This is usually the main meal of the day and is usually a hot meal. This may be prepared from fresh ingredients or a chilled or frozen meal heated in a microwave oven, or a combination of convenience and fresh ingredients such as a curry prepared with fresh meat and a jar of cook-in sauce.

This meal should include large portions of starchy carbohydrates such as potatoes, rice, pasta, couscous, noodles, bread including naan breads and other starchy vegetables such as yam.

Plenty of vegetables or salad should accompany this meal so as to contribute to the five potions of fruit and vegetables per day advocated. Casseroles, curries and stir-fries can all have extra vegetables added.

Vegetables can be fresh, frozen or canned. Frozen vegetables often have more vitamin C than fresh ones as they are frozen rapidly after picking.

Nowadays puddings are likely to be items such as fruit, ice cream, yoghurts, mousses and jellies. Fresh fruit or that canned in juice is a preferable choice to fruit canned in syrup. Low sugar and low-fat yoghurts and mousses can be chosen as can sugar-free jellies.

While baked puddings served with custard are often popular they can be time-consuming to prepare. Also they can be rich in fat and sugar.

Examples of more healthy options for puddings are:

♦ stewed fruit;
♦ crumbles made with a lot of fruit and extra oats added to the crumble mix;
♦ summer puddings made with bread and fruit;
♦ rice puddings made with skimmed or semi-skimmed milk;
♦ blancmanges or mousses made with skimmed or semi-skimmed milk;
♦ fruit charlottes topped with breadcrumbs;
♦ fruit cobblers with a thick layer of fruit topped with scone mix;
♦ scones made with low fat spread;
♦ carrot and passion cakes; and
♦ bread and butter pudding using low fat spread and lots of dried fruit.

Snacks

Between meal snacks can be useful for those working long hours and for growing children. Elderly people may benefit from snacks as their appetite for meals may be reduced.

While sweets and sugary salty snacks may be popular there is a whole range of more healthy ones. These include:

- all types of fresh fruit;
- bread and sandwiches;
- plain biscuits such as oat biscuits and digestive biscuits;
- breadsticks;
- rice snacks and rice cakes;
- oat and museli bars;
- bread buns and currant buns;
- popcorn; and
- yoghurt.

Sweets are best eaten at mealtimes for preventing the formation of acid and the resultant tooth decay.

PRINCIPLES OF A HEALTHY BALANCED MENU

When planning meals for whatever age group it is important to bear in mind the following points:

- regular meals should be provided;
- snacks are needed for growing children, those working long hours, elderly people, sportspeople, those who have been ill and those in very active occupations such as builders;
- all meals should contain a starchy carbohydrate;
- five portions of fruit and vegetables should be provided;
- a variety of foods should be included;
- meals should consist of a main part and a dessert;
- sandwiches or snack meals should also be accompanied by fruit or yoghurt or a plain bun;
- low-fat cooking methods should be promoted;
- sugar-reduced items should be included with a source of calcium and iron being provided;
- full cream milk should be included for children under two years of age;
- fish should be included three times per week;
- any meals should be appropriate for the group that is being catered for, for example, a sportswoman would have a very different diet from an elderly inactive woman; and
- 2 litres of fluid should be included each day.

Stores

Individual people, families and caterers are often recommended to have some sort of food store to tide them over a few days and prevent having to shop on a daily basis. For the caterer the store may consist of several large freezers, chilled cabinets and dry goods store.

In the domestic situation the food store may consist of a freezer containing items such as:

- frozen vegetables;
- meat;
- puddings;
- milk.

- ready-meals;
- fish;
- bread; and

A refrigerator may contain such items as:
- cheese;
- fresh meat;
- eggs;
- fruit; and

- cooked meat;
- chilled meals;
- milk;
- vegetables.

A fruit bowl will have a selection of fruit and a vegetable basket contain potatoes and other vegetables.

The bread bin may contain rolls and the biscuit and cake tins may contain biscuits, cakes and scones.

A cupboard may contain dry and canned goods such as:
- flour;
- pasta;
- canned fruit;
- oil;
- crispbreads;
- longlife UHT milk;
- jam and honey;
- sugar; and

- rice;
- canned vegetables;
- canned soups;
- packets of biscuits;
- breakfast cereal;
- evaporated milk;
- cans of oily fish such as sardines;
- jellies.

Obviously stores may vary according to the family and their budget.

An elderly person or student may have a good dry store predominating and containing items such as canned and dry products while a professional couple may have a fridge brimming full of chilled meals which they can heat in a microwave oven when they return home after working long hours.

Food labels

Food labels are a source of information on the energy values of food and the Food Labelling Regulations (1996) state that this must be provided first in kilojoules. This information is stated per 100g of food (see page 118). Caterers may be more interested in the energy value of a portion of a food so that they can enhance the energy content of menus.

Many recipes in women's magazines and also for catering provide information on the energy content of their recipes.

The calculations of energy contents of dishes are usually undertaken by nutritionists using a computer database of the 'Composition of Foods' (1991). This provides the energy content, as well as carbohydrate, fat and protein content of foods.

Question to determine progress

Discuss the value of starchy carbohydrate foods and suggest three dishes including them.
See answer in the appendix.

12 Factors affecting the British diet

Food trends

There have been a number of food issues that have affected the dietary intake of the British population. These include:

1. healthy eating;
2. heartbeat award and other awards;
3. health foods;
4. food intolerances;
5. vegetarianism and veganism;;
6. dietary supplements;
7. therapeutic diets;
8. convenience;
9. fast foods;
10. snack foods;
11. organically grown foods;
12. food labelling;
13. food additives;
14. UK ethnic minority groups;
15. international cuisine;
16. ethical considerations;
17. sport; and
18. regulations.

1. Healthy eating

Good nutrition is vital for health and the following is a summary of nutritional requirements.

Like all working machines, the body needs a supply of energy. Energy is expressed in kilojoules (kJ) but was previously expressed in calories (1 kilocalorie kcal) = 4.184 kJ).

Energy is derived from nutrients in food:

- 1g carbohydrate = 16 kJ (or 3.75 kcal);
- 1g protein = 17 kJ (or 4 kcal);
- 1g fat = 37 kJ (or 9 kcal); and
- 1g alcohol = 29 kJ (or 7 kcal).

The recommendations for the average proportion of energy in an adult's diet that should come from fat, protein and carbohydrate are:

- 35% of total energy should come from fat with 10% should come from saturates;
- 45% should come from carbohydrate foods (mainly starchy foods);
- protein intake averages 15% of total energy intake; and
- alcohol (if taken) should contribute on average around 5% of energy intake.

These figures are intended as population averages, not as targets for individuals. They refer to the habitual diet, so do not need to be met on a daily basis and certainly not by individual meals.

There are two main types of carbohydrate namely, sugar and starch. Both types provide the same amount of energy and less than half the amount provided by fat, gram for gram. At least half of the energy in the diet should come from carbohydrate, mostly from starchy foods such as bread, pasta, rice, noodles, couscous and yam.

Sugars are naturally found in milk, honey and fruit but are also added to many prepared foods (e.g. biscuits, puddings, sweets and soft drinks). Frequent consumption of these added sugars has been linked to dental decay, particularly where dental hygiene is poor.

Dietary fibre or non-starch polysaccharide (NSP) is a mixture of substances found in plant foods. Most people in the UK consume less fibre than is recommended (experts suggest 18g each day while the average person consumes only around 12g). Good sources include wholegrain cereals and breads, rice, pulses, vegetables, fruit and nuts.

Insoluble fibre helps to keep the digestive system working properly and helps to prevent bowel disorders such as constipation. Soluble fibre found in pulses, oatmeal, vegetables and fruit is thought to be particularly helpful with regard to blood cholesterol levels, when eaten as part of a low fat diet.

Protein is essential for the growth and repair of body tissues and is also a source of energy. Sources of animal protein include fish, meat, eggs, milk and cheese while sources of vegetable protein include pulses (peas, beans, lentils) nuts and cereals. Processed vegetable proteins are tofu, soya and mycoprotein.

As shown by the energy value of nutrients, fat is the most concentrated source of energy. It can be stored in the body in adipose tissue and is needed for health but in small amounts. Experts generally agree that many people in the UK are eating too much fat. This may contribute to the high rates of being overweight and obesity, which is now a serious public health problem. A high fat diet may also increase the risk of heart disease, by increasing levels of blood cholesterol.

Fats are made up of fatty acids, of which there are three main types:
♦ saturates;
♦ monounsaturates; and
♦ polyunsaturates.

Vitamins and minerals are only needed in minute amounts but are required for many processes in the body. Since the body cannot make vitamins and minerals they must be provided by the diet. Deficiency of any of these nutrients can result in ill health.

The table below gives the main functions and sources of each vitamin.

VITAMIN	MAIN FUNCTIONS	SOURCES
Fat soluble vitamins (these vitamins are provided by fat-containing foods)		
A Retinol	Maintains and repairs tissues needed for growth and development. Essential for immune function, normal and night vision.	Retinol: milk, cheese, eggs, liver, oily fish. Beta-carotene (this is a precursor for vitamin A): vegetables and fruit, especially carrots, tomatoes, mangoes, apricots and leafy green vegetables.
D Cholecalciferol	Promotes calcium and phosphate absorption from food. Essential for bones and teeth.	Sunshine, fortified margarines and breakfast cereals, oily fish and eggs.
E Tocopherol	Acts as an antioxidant, protects cell membranes from damage by oxygen.	Vegetable oils, margarines, wholegrain cereals, nuts and leafy green vegetables.
K	Essential for blood clotting.	Dark leafy green vegetables, fruit, vegetable oils, cereals and meat.
Water-soluble vitamins		
C Ascorbic Acid	Needed for the production of collagen, which is used in the structure of connective tissue and bones. Helps wound healing and iron absorption. Acts as an antioxidant.	Fruits, especially citrus fruits, fruit juices, green vegetables and potatoes.
B$_1$ Thiamin	Involved in the release of energy from carbohydrate. Important for brain and nerves.	Cereals, nuts, pulses, green vegetables, pork, fruits and fortified breakfast cereals.
B$_2$ Riboflavin	Involved in energy release, especially from fat and protein.	Liver, milk, cheese, yoghurt, eggs, green vegetables, yeast extract and fortified breakfast cereals.
B$_3$ Niacin	Involved in the release of energy.	Liver, beef, pork, lamb, fish, fortified breakfast cereals and other cereal products.
B$_{12}$ Cobalamin	Necessary for the proper formation of blood cells and nerve fibres.	Offal, meat, eggs, fish, milk, fortified breakfast cereals. No plant foods contain bioavailable B$_{12}$ naturally.
Folate	Involved in the formation of blood cells. Reduces risk of neural tube defects in early pregnancy.	Liver, orange juice, dark green vegetables, nuts, wholemeal bread and fortified breakfast cereals.
B$_6$ Pyridoxine	Involved in the metabolism of protein.	Widely distributed in foods: potatoes, beef, fish, chicken and cereals.

The table below gives the main functions and sources of each mineral.

MINERAL	MAIN FUNCTIONS	SOURCES
Calcium	Has a structural role in bones and teeth. Also essential for blood clotting, nerve and muscle impulses.	Milk and milk products, bread, pulses, green vegetables, dried fruits, nuts, seeds, soft bones found in canned fish.
Magnesium	Involved in skeletal development, nerve and muscle function. It is also necessary for the functioning of some enzymes involved in energy utilization.	Cereals, particularly wholegrain and wholemeal products, nuts, seeds, green vegetables, milk, meat and potatoes.
Phosphorus	Has a structural role in bones and teeth. Also a constituent of all the major classes of biochemical substances in the body.	Milk, milk products, bread, meat and poultry.
Sodium	Involved in maintaining the water balance of the body and is also essential for muscle and nerve activity. However, a high sodium intake has been linked to increased blood pressure.	Processed foods: bread, cereal products, breakfast cereals, meat products, pickles, canned vegetables, sauces and soups, packet snack foods, spreading fats, cheese and salt added to food.
Potassium	Complements the action of sodium.	Vegetables, potatoes, fruit (especially bananas), juices, bread, fish, nuts and seeds.
Iron	Important for the formation of red blood cells. Iron is an important component of haemoglobin the red colouring matter in red blood cells. Haemoglobin is responsible for carrying oxygen in the blood from the lungs to all cells of the body. A lack of iron can result in iron deficiency anaemia with symptoms of tiredness.	Meat and meat products are a rich source of well-absorbed iron. Plant sources are cereals, bread, breakfast cereals, leafy green vegetables, beans, lentils and dried fruit. To help absorption from plant sources, a source of vitamin C should be consumed at the same meal as the iron-containing food.
Zinc	Involved in the metabolism of protein, carbohydrates and fats, and formation of cells in the immune system.	Meat, meat products, milk, milk products, bread, cereal products (especially wholemeal), eggs, beans, lentils, nuts, sweetcorn and rice.
Copper	A component of a number of enzymes.	Shellfish, liver, meat, bread, cereal products and vegetables.

MINERAL	MAIN FUNCTIONS	SOURCES
Selenium	Acts as an antioxidant by being an integral part of one of the enzymes that protects against oxidative damage.	Nuts (especially Brazil nuts), cereals, meat and fish.
Iodine	Forms part of the thyroid hormones that help control metabolic rate, cellular metabolism and integrity of connective tissue.	Fish, seaweed, milk, milk products, beer and meat products.
Fluoride	Protects against tooth decay and has a role in bone mineralization.	Fish and fluoridated water.

Encouraging healthy eating

Research shows that although many people are interested in health, when they eat out, their main priority is still good value. Despite the growing interest in diet and health, to some people the term 'healthy' can read 'tasteless' and 'boring'. Therefore any 'healthier' items must be perceived to be enjoyable in order to be eaten. Descriptions such as 'tasty' or 'freshly cooked' may generate greater interest than descriptions such as 'low in fat' or 'the healthier option'.

Ways that the concept of healthier eating can be promoted include:

♦ adjusting the proportions of the components of the main dish to improve the balance, e.g. serving more starchy foods (such as pasta or rice) and slightly less sauce;

♦ providing bread with main meals;

♦ offering plenty of vegetables or salad;

♦ offering dressing-free side salads to accompany hot main meals;

♦ offering plenty of fresh fruit, as well as lower fat fruit-based desserts;

♦ providing smaller serving utensils and dishes for higher fat foods, e.g. smaller ladles and bowls for creamy soups;

♦ serving vegetables unglazed and items such as bread, rolls, toast, fruit breads and baked potatoes unbuttered, and by offering a choice of butter, unsaturated margarines or low fat spread separately for those customers who want them;

♦ allowing customers to add their own sauces and dressings, and highlighting healthier alternatives, for example 'fat-free' dressings;

♦ letting customers add their own cream or other toppings to desserts and by providing a choice of lower fat alternatives (e.g. 'half' fat or 'light' creams, reduced fat crème fraîche, low fat fromage frais), although portion control and cost must be considered;

♦ limiting salt addition during cooking (e.g. chips) and letting customers add their own salt or 'low sodium' alternative at the table; and

♦ posters, advertising and leaflets about healthy eating can be effective, particularly in larger catering establishments. Other promotional opportunities include theme days, free tastings and healthier catering awards.

2. Heartbeat award and other healthy eating awards

There are a number of awards related to nutrition and health, some are national while others may be organised locally by dietetic departments.

The 'Heartbeat Award' is a national award and was developed by the Health Education Authority and Department of Health and is endorsed by the Chartered Institute of Environmental Health. It is a nationally recognised award given to caterers who are committed to offering greater choice to customers, through the provision of a healthy environment and healthier food choices. It is aimed at all catering establishments including workplace, school

THE HEARTBEAT AWARD

- **Developed by the Health Education Authority and Department of Health and is endorsed by the Chartered Institute of Environmental Health**

- **A nationally recognised award given to caterers who are committed to offering greater choice to customers, through the provision of a healthy environment and healthier food choices**

- **Aimed at all catering establishments including workplace, school and hospital canteens, sandwich bars, pubs, hotels and restaurants**

- **Recognises caterers' commitment to promoting good health and provides good publicity**

- **Environmental Health Department**

AWARDS

- **Heartbeat Award**
- **Healthy Schools' Award**
- **Healthy Workplace Initiatives**
- **Local Awards**
- **School Cook of the Year**
- **Care Cook**
- **Various other awards for culinary work**

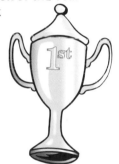

and hospital canteens, sandwich bars, pubs, hotels and restaurants. The award recognises caterers' commitment to promoting good health and provides good publicity.

Other awards such as the 'healthy schools' award' have a component on nutrition that the school can choose to apply for.

3. Health foods

There are no good or bad foods but well-balanced or poorly-balanced diets. While there are some foods that we should not eat too much of, or eat too often, there are many foods that we should be increasing in the diet, such as fruit and vegetables, starchy food and oily fish.

Eating is about enjoyment and all foods can be included in a healthy diet, as long as the right balance is achieved. The Balance of Good Health provides a pictorial representation of the overall balance of a healthy diet.

All foods have some type of nutritional content and therefore an impact on health.

Health food shops often stock a range of unusual foods such as may be useful for people following a gluten-free diet or a milk-free diet. Such foods as milk- and gluten-free foods can usually be purchased from supermarkets but there may be a wider variety in health food shops.

Often products for sale in health food shops may be more expensive than those found in supermarkets but they may be useful as treats.

Additionally health food shops may sell a number of supplements. Again these may be useful but a new group of foods has been developed over the last few years, termed 'functional foods'. Such foods have heath benefits in additions to their nutritional benefits.

Examples of such foods are:

♦   special spreads which contain plant stanols to lower blood cholesterol levels;
♦   probiotic drinks which have specially cultured bacteria in them to promote bowel health; and
♦   breads which contain phyto-oestrogens for health of post-menopausal women.

Any claims relating to functional foods must be carefully worded and based on research.

4. Food intolerances

Food intolerances are adverse reactions to food and food allergies are part of this group. More people believe themselves to be intolerant or allergic to foods than is actually the case. But the possibility of food allergy or an intolerance to a food should always be taken seriously because it can cause severe, possibly life-threatening, reactions and chronic ill health. Food intolerance is an umbrella term covering a wide range of unpleasant reactions to food or food components. It can result in symptoms such as abdominal pain, diarrhoea, headaches, migraine, fatigue, asthma or a skin reaction, but these symptoms can also occur for reasons unrelated to food. Food allergy is a specific form of food intolerance in which the reaction provoked involves the body's immune system.

Many foods can provoke adverse reactions but the most common triggers of reactions are foods such as peanuts and milk (see page 90 for the full list of foods causing intolerances).

The response can be so severe that it can be fatal if untreated. Nuts, shellfish and sesame seeds are the most common triggers of a very severe, life-threatening reaction (anaphylaxis). In Britain there are about six reported deaths each year due to food-induced anaphylaxis, most of which are triggered by food eaten out of the home.

Any or all of the following symptoms may occur in anyone with a food intolerance:

♦   swelling of the throat and mouth;
♦   difficulty swallowing or speaking;
♦   difficulty breathing;
♦   skin rash or flushing;
♦   abdominal cramps, nausea, vomiting;
♦   sudden feeling of weakness (drop in blood pressure); and
♦   collapse and unconsciousness.

Someone diagnosed as having a food allergy will need to ensure that all possible sources of the problem food are avoided. For some people with nut allergy even minute quantities can have rapid and fatal effects. If nuts or nut oils are used in a recipe and their presence is not clear from the name of the food, or its presentation, the dish should be labelled. It is essential that suppliers provide accurate written details about all the allergen-containing ingredients in prepared meals and pre-packaged food.

5. Vegetarianism and veganism

About 3% of the population is truly vegetarian. Many people claim to be vegetarian but are not totally strict.

A well-planned vegetarian diet can be a very healthy one but, as with any diet, it must contain the right balance of foods. Vegetable-based dishes are not always healthier choices if they are made with a lot of oil, pastry, cheese or creamy sauces and it is important for caterers to offer lower-fat vegetarian choices (e.g. vegetable and bean casserole, nut risotto).

Strictly speaking, vegetarians do not eat meat or fish but the term 'vegetarianism' can mean a variety of different things and the types of foods restricted can vary enormously.

Vegans usually exclude any animal-derived ingredients added to manufactured food, such as emulsifiers derived from animal fats (e.g. lecithin) and firming agents (e.g. gelatine). Products which are seen to involve the exploitation of animals (e.g. honey) or which have undergone safety testing using animals, may also be avoided. Catering for vegans not only requires consideration about the ingredients used, the foods must also not come into contact with any animal products during preparation or service.

Because many foods are restricted, vegan diets require careful consideration to ensure that they provide sufficient protein, vitamins and minerals.

Avoidance of dairy products can increase the risk of low intakes of calcium, vitamin B_2 and vitamin B_{12}. Vegans are at higher risk of iron and zinc deficiency.

Alternative sources of these nutrients are:

♦ cereals, soya products, pulses and nuts for protein;
♦ bread, green vegetables, pulses, nuts, tempeh and soya mince for calcium;
♦ fortified foods, leafy green vegetables, wholegrain breads and breakfast cereals for vitamin B_2;
♦ fortified foods, for example breakfast cereals or some vegetable extract spreads for vitamin B_{12};
♦ fortified breakfast cereals, pulses and legumes, green vegetables, bread, nuts and dried fruit for iron - serving fruit or fruit juice containing vitamin C (e.g. citrus fruits) with a meal can improve the amount of iron absorbed from foods of plant origin; and
♦ cereals, pulses and nuts for zinc.

The high fibre content of starchy foods, pulses, fruit and vegetables can make a vegetarian diet very bulky and it may be difficult for children and others with small appetites to eat sufficient to meet their energy and nutrient needs. Whole milk, full fat dairy products, soya products and fortified breakfast cereals are important foods for young children adopting a vegetarian diet.

6. Dietary supplements

Supplements can be useful for certain groups of people who have special needs. For example, vitamin drops are recommended for children from six months to two years, elderly or housebound people may benefit from a vitamin D supplement and women are advised to take folic acid supplements if they are planning to have a baby and until the end of the twelfth week of pregnancy.

SUPPLEMENTS

- **Cannot make up for a poor diet**
- **Supplements useful for certain groups**
  - **Children aged 6 months to 2 years**
    Vitamin drops
  - **Elderly or housebound people**
    Vitamin D
  - **Women planning a pregnancy/pregnant**
    Folic acid
  - **Vegans**
    Vitamin B_{12}

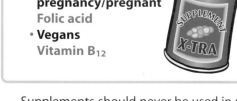

VITAMIN AND MINERAL SUPPLEMENTS

- **Infants and children**
- **Those on restricted diets**
- **Elderly people**
- **Pregnant women**
- **Alcoholics**
- **Strict vegetarians (i.e. vegans)**
- **Some ethnic groups (e.g. Asians)**
- **People on low incomes**
- **Women with heavy periods**
- **Post-menopausal women**

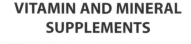

Supplements should never be used in place of a balanced diet. In addition, just because a little of a vitamin is good for you, it does not mean that much more is better. Some minerals compete with each other for absorption, e.g. high doses of iron can reduce absorption of zinc. This can cause problems In people who are marginally deficient in these nutrients. Also, some vitamins and minerals have adverse effects at very high levels (e.g. vitamin A, selenium).

7. Therapeutic diets

Some people require to adjust what they eat to deal with a medical problem. This includes catering for people with coeliac disease, diabetes, obesity, those with raised lipid levels, pancreatic disorders, metabolic condition and food intolerances (see Chapter 9).

8. Convenience

Nowadays people often have minimal time for food preparation and thus convenience foods can be invaluable. Such food needs minimal preparation and can be frozen, canned, chilled or dehydrated.

Sometimes the only preparation required is heating in a microwave oven. It is important that the instructions are followed and the food is correctly heated.

This type of food when in the form of complete meals can be invaluable in contributing to the diet but can be high in fat, salt, sugar and food additives and also low in fruit and vegetable levels. It is easy to improve

CONVENIENCE FOODS

Processed or partly-prepared by food manufacturer

May be ready-to-eat or need minimal preparation e.g. just heating

Popular due to:
- **Less leisure time**
- **Working women**
- **Increased ownership of freezers and microwaves**
- **Influence of advertising**

May be high in fat

Low in fruit and vegetables

Higher level of additives e.g. preservatives

May not be correctly heated/prepared

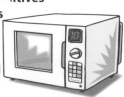

the balance of a ready-prepared meal by adding extra vegetables such as frozen ones or adding extra carbohydrate as bread, pasta or rice.

Convenience foods can be extremely useful for those living on their own.

9. Fast foods

Like convenience foods, fast foods are helpful to those who have limited time for shopping, preparing, cooking and eating foods.

Such foods can be low in fruit and vegetable content and high in fat and salt. Also the sugar content of milk shakes and other drinks and desserts may be high.

Many of the fast foods are designed to be eaten quickly and easily eaten from the hand.

Due to the large number of fast food outlets there is a tremendous variety of foods on offer. Often these appeal greatly to children due to the promotional gifts and foods that are provided for children.

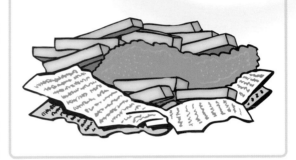

FAST FOODS AND SNACK FOODS

- **Takeaways**
    - **May be high in salt and sugar**
    - **Snacks can be used as part of a diet**

Many of the fast foods are reasonably priced, quickly and efficiently served and are of a consistent quality.

There is no reason why fast foods cannot be part of a varied diet. An unbalanced diet could result if the total diet was based on such foods with little extra fruit and vegetables.

Some caution should be exercised in the choice of items, with French fries and deep fried battered foods being an occasional treat rather than a regular feature of an intake.

10. Snack foods

Snacks can be useful for all types of diet. They are particularly useful for growing children, teenagers, those with long working hours and gaps between meals, elderly people who have small appetites, those who have been ill and require extra protein and energy from their diet, pregnant women, women who are breastfeeding, and those who are expending a high level of energy, such as those working in manual labour, e.g. builders and sportsmen and women.

Sensible snacks can be based on:

- fruit of all types both fresh and dried;
- bread made into sandwiches and as toast;
- bagels;
- milk and milky drinks such as malted milk;
- smoothies;
- yoghurts;
- plain biscuits;
- crispbreads;
- breadsticks;
- breakfast cereals;

♦   currant buns; and
♦   plain scones.

Some snacks are high in fat, sugar and salt and caution should be exercised about not eating too many of these. Sweet and sugary items are best taken with meals to prevent accelerating dental decay.

Young children can fill up on such snacks as packets of savoury snacks and, as a result, have little appetite for main meals.

11. Organically grown foods

To enhance growth and prevent attack by pests, many crops are grown with the use of agrochemicals such as fertilisers and pesticides. Also animals may be reared in environments where frequent use of antibiotics is required.

Some people prefer to only eat foods grown organically without the use of such agrochemicals and animals reared by traditional husbandry methods.

Such organic foods are grown to set standards and are accredited by organisations such as the Soil Association. For a farmer to move from the usual type of farming in use in this country whereby agrochemicals are used to an organic type of farming can take several years as the residues of chemicals need to be given time to be lost from the soil.

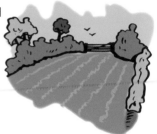

ORGANIC FOODS

• **Grown without agrochemicals**
• **Reared without chemicals**
• **Most imported**
• **No nutritional differences**

For the organic standard to be achieved crops must not be grown near those which are genetically modified.

Organically grown fruit and vegetables usually take longer to grow than those grown with pesticides and fertilisers which can promote growth. Different varieties of crops tend to be grown organically so there may be slight flavour differences between organic and non-organically grown food.

There is however no real nutritional difference between organic and non-organically grown food.

Organically grown food is widely available in supermarkets these days and tends to be more expensive. Due to difficulties in meeting customer demands for such foods some 90% of organic food is imported. Even if it is imported it is still grown to the same standards and this is carefully checked by the major buyers of foods in supermarkets.

12. Food labelling

Nutrition information is not required by law for any products, unless a nutritional claim is made (such as 'low in fat'). Food labels are a source of information on the energy values of food and the Food Labelling Regulations (1984) state that this must be provided first in kilojoules. This is stated per 100g of food. Where labelling is used, UK and EU laws and guidelines dictate the format. At a minimum, the information provided should list the nutrients known as the 'Big 4'.

FOOD LABELS

The 'BIG 4':
- **Energy – in kilojoules (kJ) or kilocalories (kcal)**
- **Protein – in grams (g)**
- **Carbohydrate – in grams (g)**
- **Fat – in grams (g)**

The 'BIG 4' and the 'LITTLE 4':
- **Energy – in kilojoules (kJ) or kilocalories (kcal)**
- **Protein – in grams (g)**
- **Carbohydrate – in grams (g)**
  - **of which sugars – in grams (g)**
- **Fat – in grams (g)**
  - **of which saturates – in grams (g)**
- **Fibre – in grams (g)**
- **Sodium – in grams (g)**

FOOD LABELS

Must provide:
- **Name of food**
- **Ingredients**
- **Durability**
- **Manufacturer**
- **Nutritional content (Per 100g) if claim made**
- **Energy**
- **Protein**
- **Carbohydrate**
- **Fat**

Claims
- **To describe an item as 'low fat' it must contain no more than 3g of fat per 100g of food (or per 100ml for liquids)**

- **A 'reduced fat' food should contain at least 25% less fat than a comparable food**

- **A 'low salt' food must contain no more than 40mg of sodium per 100g**

The 'Big 4' is as follows:
- Energy – in kilojoules (kJ) or kilocalories (kcal);
- Protein – in grams (g);
- Carbohydrate – in grams (g); and
- Fat – in grams (g).

More detailed information can be provided by listing the 'Little 4' (sugars, saturates, fibre and sodium), as well as the 'Big 4'. The 'Big 4' and the 'Little 4':
- Energy – in kilojoules (kJ) or kilocalories (kcal);
- Protein – in grams (g);
- Carbohydrate – in grams (g);
  - of which sugars – in grams (g);
- Fat – in grams (g);
  - of which saturates – in grams (g);
- Fibre – in grams (g); and
- Sodium – in grams (g).

Other nutrients, such as monounsaturates, cholesterol or starch, can be declared. Which format is chosen will depend on the health claim, e.g. if a claim is made relating to the content of sugars, fibre or sodium, both the 'Big 4' and 'little 4' must be listed. All information must be given per 100 grams (or 100ml) of the edible portion of the food. Information can also be given per serving or per portion, provided that the number of portions is stated. The rules governing labelling of vitamins and minerals are more complex.

For each vitamin or mineral the amount present can only be listed if the food provides a significant proportion of the Recommended Daily Allowance (RDA), as defined by European legislation.

Labelling of Genetically Modified (GM) Foods is required and caterers are legally required to label foods that contain GM soya or maize and any GM additives and flavourings.

The information must be provided either on a label attached to the food, on a menu or notice or verbally via serving staff.

The Trading Standards or Environmental Health Departments at Local Authorities are responsible for enforcing the labelling requirements. It is anticipated that they will check for compliance in the course of their routine inspections. Businesses are required to take reasonable steps and exercise due diligence to ensure that they comply with the requirements.

Guideline Daily Amounts (GDAs) are seen on some food labels. These are the average amounts of energy, fat and sodium that are needed by the body each day.

A TYPICAL FOOD LABEL

Typical values per
serving per 100g

Energy 1260 kJ/300 kcal
Protein 20.4g
Carbohydrate 42.5g
of which: sugars 7.8g
Fat 42.5g
of which: saturates 1.7g
Fibre 2.7g
Sodium 0.7g

13. Food additives

To enable most of the foods that we eat today to be manufactured, food additives are important, especially for fast foods, convenience foods and snacks.

Margarine could not be produced without emulsifiers and stabilizers to keep the water and fat together. If there were no additives present many foods would have much reduced shelf-lives and some foods may become hazardous. Additives are also used to provide food with characteristic flavours, colours and textures. The term additive is a broad one and covers such products as preservatives, antioxidants, colourings, emulsifiers and stabilizers and artificial sweeteners. Perhaps the group of food additives we come across most are the preservatives. These compounds can help reduce food wastage, give a wider choice of foods and help to keep food safe. Most responsible food companies have a policy as regards the use of food additives to make use of them only when they are technically necessary, and where

FOOD ADDITIVES

- **Use of food additives**
  - **Ready-prepared foods**
  - **Consistent final product**
  - **Essential uses**
  - **E numbers signify that an additive is approved for use in the European Community**
  - **It is approved for use only in certain foods in set maximum amounts**
  - **Food labels are required to include the ingredients in a food**

- **Occasional intolerance to food additives**
  - **Children with hyperactivity**
  - **ADHD (attention deficit hyperactivity disorder)**
  - **Asthma and skin conditions**

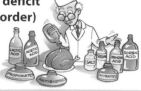

possible to use natural additives, for example, vitamin E as an antioxidant, in preference to synthetic additives.

All of the compounds allowed in food are tabulated on permitted lists, and often the maximum amount of the additive allowed is also specified. They have all had a good deal of research carried out on their safety and many continue to be studied to make sure that they are safe. A few people are allergic to some food additives, for example, some children are allergic to the colour tartrazine, but in the main the amount of additive used in a product causes no problem. Perhaps the potential problems lie in the effects of combined additives. If a person consumes a variety of foods, they may take in a whole range of different additives and the long-term effects of this are less well understood. This is one of the reasons that many manufacturers have decided to limit the use of additives.

Approved food additives usually have a special number. Any number that also has an E designation means that the additive has been approved by the European Community. The purity of the additive is also described in EC legislation. If an additive is present in food it must be declared on the label of the packaged product. The additive may be properly named, for example, ascorbic acid (vitamin C) or may be listed by its code number E300.

14. UK ethnic minority groups

A large number of ethnic minority groups now live in the UK, the largest being the Asian. However, even within an ethnic minority group, the types of food chosen can vary widely. The traditional diets of most ethnic minority groups contain a large amount of starchy foods (such as cereals, rice, cassava, yams, potatoes), pulses, vegetables and fruit, and are likely to be beneficial in terms of health. Although older members of ethnic minority groups often maintain their traditional dietary patterns in Britain, many younger people, particularly those born in this country, are increasingly adopting Western style food habits.

RELIGIOUS GROUP	FOODS AND DRINKS WHICH MAY BE AVOIDED
Muslim	Pork, non-halal meat and chicken, shellfish, alcohol
Hindu	Meat (some eat lamb and chicken), fish (some eat white fish), eggs, alcohol
Sikh	Beef, pork (some are vegetarian), alcohol
Buddhist	Chicken, lamb, pork, beef, shellfish (some avoid all fish), alcohol
Rastafarian	Animal products (except milk), foods which are not Ital (i.e. avoid tinned or processed food), alcohol, tea, coffee
Jewish	Pork, meat which is not kosher, shellfish Meat and milk products must not be served at the same meal or cooked together

15. International cuisine

With continental travel on holidays and business as well as exposure to numerous different cuisines from those of different ethnic groups, the United Kingdom now has a population enjoying different types of cooking. Items such as Indian curries, Chinese stir-fries, American hamburgers, Italian pizzas and pasta dishes are all now familiar adjuncts to traditional United Kingdom fare.

16. Ethical considerations

Ethical considerations are to the fore for those who follow vegetarian and vegan diets. Those who choose organic food often do so for ethical and environmental issues of animal welfare and environmental considerations of use of chemicals.

17. Sport

For those who take part in active sports fluid is vital.

Carbohydrate should provide the main source of energy for sports people. Regular snacks of starchy carbohydrates are advocated both before and after the main activities.

Many sports people mistakenly feel they should take massive amounts of protein. Such a high protein intake can be damaging to the kidneys.

19. Regulations

These regulations on food and nutrition include a number of laws on food including those on food labelling. There are also 'The National Nutritional Standards for School Lunches', which were published in 2000 by the Department for Education and Employment.

FOODS AND DRINKS

Milk and milk products

Most milk in this country is consumed as pasteurised semi-skimmed milk. To pasteurise or sterilise milk, the milk is heated before bottling or putting into cartons.

Milk is also dried by heating it. This milk may be skimmed or full fat. Some skimmed milks are dried and then have the fat replaced by adding unsaturated oil to it.

Butter is made from the cream which is the fat in milk. This cream floats to the top of the milk and is removed and churned to cause the fat to coagulate and form butter. Salt is traditionally added and the butter worked to form the spreadable product.

Cheese is made by coagulating the milk protein with rennet (traditionally rennet was obtained from the stomach of calves, but most rennet now is from vegetarian sources). This milk protein is brought together as a firm curd leaving the liquid whey which contains most of

---

MILK AND MILK PRODUCTS

- **Dried milk**

- **Yoghurts**
  - **Bacterial culture**

- **Cheese**
  - **Cheese is hardened by adding rennet - milk protein casein coagulates**

- **Cheddar approx**
  - **33% fat**
  - **33% water**
  - **33% protein**

Exposure to sunlight destroys riboflavin and vitamin C in milk

- **Butter made from cream**
  - **fat at top of milk**
  - **vitamin A and D**

MILK AND MILK PRODUCTS

- **Cows' milk**

- **Consumption approx. 280ml/half pint per day**

  - **Whole fat 3.98% fat**
  - **Semi-skimmed 1.6% fat**
  - **Skimmed 0.1% fat**

- **Semi-skimmed most popular**

- **Children under 2 years - whole milk**
Can introduce semi-skimmed at 2 years
Can introduce skimmed milk at 5 years

- **Cream - contains vitamin A and D**

Most milk pasteurised – heat 72°C for 15 seconds

Sterilised – heat 110°C for 20-30 minutes

the lactose found in milk and water. The curd is pressed to make it firm and form the hard cheese such as cheddar.

The pasteurisation, sterilisation and drying of milk as well as making butter and cheese are all commercial processes. The most popular milk is semi-skimmed milk which contains 1.6% fat. Homogenised milk has the cream (fat) dispersed throughout the milk.

Sugars

Sugar gives a well-liked flavour to many foods and drinks and is an essential ingredient of such items as sweets, chocolate, cakes, pastries and puddings as well as being added to teas and coffees and also breakfast cereals.

Table sugar is the disaccharide technically called sucrose.

Honey contains about 75% of the total amount of sugar contained in white granulated sugar but it is not considered to be a good source of any other nutrients. It is slightly sweeter than refined sugar, so smaller amounts can be used in place of sugar in some recipes. However, it should not be eaten too frequently as it can contribute to tooth decay.

Puddings

All types of puddings and cakes contain sugar as one of the essential ingredients. Puddings and cakes can be very tempting to those with a small appetite. The choice of thick and creamy yoghurt rather than a low fat one can provide four times as many calories.

Calorie values of puddings per 100g are as follows:

◆	sponge pudding	340 kcal
◆	apple crumble	207 kcal
◆	treacle sponge	333 kcal
◆	milk jelly made with whole milk	88 kcal
◆	jelly made with water	61 kcal
◆	thick and creamy fruit yoghurt	399 kcal
◆	low fat fruit yoghurt	90 kcal

Unfortunately sucrose can contribute to the development of dental caries. The presence of sucrose causes the growth of bacteria in the mouth and the formation of a sticky substance called plaque where acid is formed by the bacteria. This acid then erodes the tooth enamel. It is more important to cut down on sugar in snacks than in desserts at main meals.

Although eating too much sugar can contribute towards over-consumption of energy in an unbalanced diet, the main concern relates to dental caries. But it is the frequency of sugar consumption, rather than the amount, that seems to be important in terms of dental caries risk. This is because, each time sugar is eaten, there is the potential for bacteria present in dental plaque to ferment the sugar, producing acid. It is this acid that attacks dental enamel. Current advice is to restrict the consumption of sugar-rich foods and drinks to four or five occasions per day, ideally keeping to meal times. Providing low-sugar snacks is, therefore, more important than reducing the amount of sugar in desserts, particularly for children.

Frequent consumption of sugary items can be most damaging to teeth and therefore sucking boiled sweets or sugary lollies and constantly sipping sugary drinks is more harmful than taking sugary items and sweets with or after meals.

Sweeteners

Today there is a range of sweeteners available for use instead of sugar. These can be purchased in supermarkets and chemists for use in drinks in the home and are used by manufacturers in soft drinks. Such sweeteners include cyclamates, saccharin, acesulphame and aspartame. They are all extremely sweet and thus only small amounts are needed. They do not contribute to the energy intake and thus can be used in weight loss. Also they are not detrimental to tooth health.

Intense sweeteners, such as aspartame and saccharin, are used widely in manufactured foods. Tablet, liquid and sprinkle sweeteners can also be added to drinks, on cereals or in desserts. Because they are so sweet, only small amounts need to be used. Some people are concerned about the safety of these sweeteners and the fact that they are now added to so many foods. Sweeteners, like all food additives, are only permitted for use in food after careful evaluation, which includes rigorous safety checks by scientific committees. An acceptable daily intake (ADI) is set for each additive. This is the amount that can be consumed every day over a lifetime without any appreciable health risk. Current trends show that the ADI for sweeteners is very unlikely to be regularly exceeded by most adults. However, it is important to dilute concentrated soft drinks containing saccharin for infants and young children more than for adults to avoid the risk of providing more of the sweetener than is recommended.

For those with diabetes, intense sweeteners are ideal. Such sweeteners as sorbitol and fructose are used in so-called 'diabetic products'. Such products are not recommended as they are high in calories and also have side effects on the bowel which may cause diarrhoea.

Fats

Fats are found in a number of foods. There are visible fats such as those in butter, margarine, oils and spreads and hidden fats such as in cakes, chocolate and ice cream.

Butter and margarine contain 82% and 79% fat respectively and 744kcal (3059kJ) and 388kcal (2954kJ) per 100g respectively. Adding an extra pat of butter to mashed potatoes can

UNSATURATED FATS (MONOUNSATURATED)

Monounsaturated fats are found in:
- **Olive oil**
- **Rapeseed oil**
- **Walnut oil**
- **Avocado**

Some margarines and spreads are made from monounsaturated fats

add extra fat and energy, as a 10 gram pat of butter will provide about 90 extra calories.

Butter which is made from the cream in cows' milk naturally contains vitamins A and D. Margarine for retail use must have vitamins A and D added to it.

Low fat spreads contain 40-80% fat depending on the type.

Polyunsaturated spreads have been manufactured to have a higher proportion of polyunsaturated fatty acids than butter or margarine. Other spreads are manufactured to contain a higher proportion of olive oil, which is a monounsaturated fatty acid.

Mayonnaise – the full fat variety – which is available contains about 75% fat and the low calorie varieties of mayonnaise contain about 28% fat.

Hard cheeses such as cheddar cheese contain about 35%, Brie about 29%, low fat Cheddar cheese about 16% and cottage cheese 4% fat.

Cream contains a significant amount of fat. Typical fat content of different creams and alternatives are as follows:

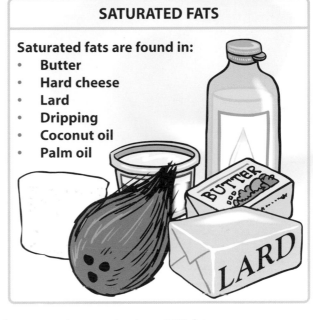

SATURATED FATS

Saturated fats are found in:
- **Butter**
- **Hard cheese**
- **Lard**
- **Dripping**
- **Coconut oil**
- **Palm oil**

Percentage fat	
♦ Jersey/clotted cream	64%
♦ Double cream	48%
♦ Crème fraîche ordinary	40%
♦ Whipping cream	39%
♦ UHT canned spray cream	32%
♦ Soured cream	20%
♦ Half-fat crème fraîche	15%
♦ Single cream	19%
♦ Half-cream	13%
♦ Quark	Trace of fat

Too much fat in the diet can contribute to obesity and increase the risk of chronic diseases, such as heart disease. Although rates have been falling, Britain still has one of the highest heart disease rates in the world and it is the most common cause of premature death.

Types of Fatty Acids	Where they are found	Effects on health
Saturates	Found largely in fats of animal origin: meat (beef, pork, lamb), meat fats (suet, lard, dripping) and dairy products (butter, milk, cream, cheese). Although all oils contain some saturates, two vegetable oils naturally contain a relatively large proportion of saturates: palm oil and coconut oil. Fats and oils rich in saturates are used in the commercial manufacture of many biscuits, pastries, cakes, pies, snacks and other baked foods.	A high intake may raise blood cholesterol levels and increase the risk of a heart attack.
Unsaturates	There are two categories of unsaturates: monounsaturates and polyunsaturates.	These fatty acids are thought to be beneficial to health if they replace saturates in the diet
Monounsaturates	Found in fats of both plant and animal origin. Olive oil and rapeseed oil are particularly rich sources. Other sources include dairy products, nuts and meat.	Used in place of saturates, these fatty acids may lower blood cholesterol and reduce the risk of heart disease.
Polyunsaturates	There are two main families of polyunsaturates: n-6 (or omega 6) and n-3 (or omega 3) fatty acids. n-6 polyunsaturates are found largely in fats of plant origin, including sunflower, soya, sesame, corn, soyabean, cottonseed and safflower oils. Wholegrain cereals (e.g. wheat, barley, oats) also contain small quantities of n-6 polyunsaturates. Some oils (e.g. walnut, rapeseed, linseed oil) and oil-rich fish (including herring, mackerel, salmon, tuna – not tinned and trout) are rich in n-3 polyunsaturates.	Both n-6 and n-3 polyunsaturates are important for health. Populations which eat large amounts of oil-rich fish have much lower rates of heart attacks and strokes.

Bread, other cereals and potatoes

Wheat is a major source of starchy carbohydrate in this country. It is made into bread, biscuits, pasta, noodles, breakfast cereals, puddings and pastries as well as being used as an ingredient to thicken soups and sauces. Wheat is turned into flour by the process of milling, where the wheat grain is passed between large rollers.

The wheat grain contains about 65-80% carbohydrate, which is in the form of starch. It also contains 7-13% protein. Wheat higher in protein levels is used for bread and pasta making. Lower protein levels in wheat are required for making flour which is to be used for biscuit and cake making.

The outer part of the wheat grain is called the husk and this contains dietary fibre or NSP. Attached to the outer husk is the wheat germ which contains most of the B vitamins. During the milling process the husk can be removed plus most of the wheat germ.

Wholemeal flour has the whole of the wheat retained in the resultant flour. White flour has only 73% of the original wheat grain retained. Thus most of the dietary fibre and calcium, B vitamins and iron are removed in white flour. Therefore iron, B vitamins of thiamin and niacin and calcium are added back to the flour.

Rice is another staple starchy carbohydrate. White rice has the outer husk removed and hence is lower in fibre than wholegrain brown rice.

The wheat grain contains about 65-80% carbohydrate which is in the form of starch. It also contains 7-13% protein. Wheat higher in protein levels is used for bread and pasta making. Lower protein levels in wheat are required for making flour which is to be sued for biscuit and cake making.

The outer part of the wheat grain is called the husk and this contains dietary fibre or NSP. Attached to the outer husk is the wheat germ which contains most of the B vitamins. During the milling process the husk can be removed plus most of the wheat germ. White flour has no remaining husk left.

Wholemeal flour has the whole of the wheat retained in the resultant flour. White flour has only 73% of the original wheat grain retained. Thus most of the dietary fibre and calcium, B vitamins and iron is removed in white flour. Therefore iron, B vitamins of thiamin and niacin and calcium is added back to the flour.

Rice is another staple starchy carbohydrate. White rice has the outer husk removed and hence is lower in fibre than wholegrain brown rice.

Food tables

Food tables are used to provide information to enable an analysis of recipes and diets to be made. Food tables have been developed after careful analysis of the range and amounts of different nutrients found in a variety of foods commonly found in the diet.

McCance and Widdowson's *The Composition of Foods*, produced originally by the Royal Society of Chemistry and the Ministry of Agriculture Fisheries and Food and now by the Food Standards Agency, is the standard source of information used in this country.

Food hygiene

It is important that all food is correctly stored and prepared.

Question to determine progress

Suggest ways in which a canteen manager can promote healthy eating. **See answer in the appendix.**

Appendix Answers to questions in each chapter.

CHAPTER 1

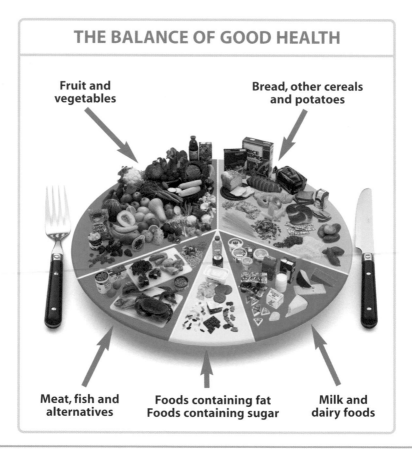

THE BALANCE OF GOOD HEALTH

Fruit and vegetables

Bread, other cereals and potatoes

Meat, fish and alternatives

Foods containing fat
Foods containing sugar

Milk and dairy foods

CHAPTER 2

a) Peer pressure
Advertising
Family habits
Finance
Time

b) Finance
Season
Availability/access
Habits
Loneliness

c) Finance
Availability/access
Convenience
Cooking facilities
Family pressures
Advertising

CHAPTER 3

- Proteins are required for growth and repair of body tissues.
- Proteins are made up of amino acids.
- Amino acids consist of essential and non-essential amino acids.
- Nitrogen is a key element in protein.

- Proteins are found in foods such as meat, fish, eggs, cheese, milk. Nuts and pulses are key vegetarian sources of protein.
- Protein tissues are found in the body in skin, vital organs, (for example, heart, lungs, intestines and liver) muscles, hair, nails, enzymes, hormones and blood cells.
- During periods of growth as occurs in children and teenagers progressively more protein is required.

CHAPTER 4

- Vitamin C (ascorbic acid) is a water-soluble vitamin. It acts as an antioxidant.
- It is needed for healing and formation of corrective tissue. It aids the absorption of non-haem iron. As an antioxidant it promotes the effect of the immune system and helps protect against coronary heart disease and cancers.
- It is found in citrus fruit, salad, vegetables, fruit, potatoes.
- Iron is found in 2 forms: haem iron and non-haem iron. It is required for the function of haemoglobin found in red blood cells. This transports oxygen from the lungs to every cell of the body. Haem iron is well absorbed. It is found in red meat and dark fish. Non-haem iron is found in pulses, cereals and vegetables; it is poorly absorbed.
- Vegetarians can be at risk of iron deficiency anaemia as can woman of child-bearing age, elderly people and toddlers.

CHAPTER 5

- Women maximum units of alcohol per week 21.
- Men maximum units of alcohol per week 28.
- Liver cirrhosis
- Obesity and the associated risk of liver disease, type 2 diabetes, strokes.

CHAPTER 6

- Digestion is the process whereby food is broken down into the compact nutrients, for example, glucose, amino acids and fatty acids.
- Absorption is the process where the nutrients pass across the intestinal wall into the bloodstream.

CHAPTER 7

- Weaning is the process when food other than milk is introduced into baby's diet.
- It should not occur before 4 months.
- Foods given should be puréed.
- Items such as puréed rice, meat, poultry, vegetables and fruits should be given.
- Citrus fruit, wheat and nuts should be avoided.

CHAPTER 8

- Malnutrition is disordered eating which results in consequences to health.
- In the UK examples of malnutrition are lack of exercise and overeating causing obesity.
- Coronary heart disease due to excessive saturated fat.
- Bowel cancer due to too little dietary fibre and antioxidants.

CHAPTER 9

♦ Avoid adding sugar to drinks and on cereals.
♦ Provide low-sugar items, for example, jellies and squashes.
♦ Reduce the fat content of the diet.
♦ Provide plenty of starchy carbohydrate foods.
♦ Provide 5 portions of fruit and vegetables per day.
♦ Ensure the diet promotes weight loss.

CHAPTER 10

Hindus do not eat beef – many are strict vegetarians.

Sample menu:
♦ BREAKFAST
   Orange juice and water
   Wholegrain cereal plus milk (full cream milk for toddler)
   Toast plus low fat spread and jam

♦ MID-MORNING
   Piece of fruit plus squash or tea (milk for toddler)

♦ LUNCH
   Sandwiches made with a filling of canned salmon and salad, apple and yoghurt (eaten at home by mother, toddler and grandmother and taken to work by father)
   Fresh juice with water, tea or coffee.

♦ MID-AFTERNOON
   Biscuit plus milk for toddler with tea for the rest of the family.

♦ EVENING MEAL
   Vegetarian curry served with rice and naan bread plus side salad. Fresh fruit salad plus ice cream. Milk for the toddler. Tea for the rest of the family.

Additional drinks or water throughout the day.

CHAPTER 11

♦ Starchy carbohydrates: provide energy.
♦ Low in fat
♦ Filling
♦ Provide B vitamins
♦ Provide fibre especially if wholegrain

Examples of meals:
♦ pasta bake
♦ risotto
♦ stir fry with noodles

CHAPTER 12

- Provide low fat, tempting dishes.
- Provide starchy carbohydrates.
- Provide plenty of fruit and vegetables.
- Provide promotions such as posters.
- Apply for healthy eating awards.

Glossary

BMR	Basal Metabolic Rate
COMA	The Committee on Medical Aspects of Food and Nutrition Policy
DoH	The Department of Health
DRV	Dietary Reference Value. The term used to cover LRNI, EAR, RNI and safe intake. See Department of Health, *Report on Health and Social Subjects: 41. Dietary Reference Values for Food Energy and Nutrients for the United Kingdom*, HMSO (London, 1991).
EAR	The Estimated Average Requirement of a group of people for energy or protein or a vitamin or mineral. About half will usually need more than the EAR, and half less.
Extrinsic sugars	Any sugar which is not contained within the cell walls of food. Examples are sugars in honey, table sugar and lactose in milk and milk products.
FSA	Food Standards Agency
Intrinsic sugars	Any sugar which is contained within the cell wall of a food.
LRNI	The Lower Reference Nutrient Intake for protein or a vitamin or mineral. An amount of nutrient that is enough for only the few people in the group who have low needs.
MAFF	The Ministry of Agriculture, Fisheries and Food
Mean	The average value
NDNS	The National Diet and Nutrition Survey
NFS	National Food Survey
NMES	Non-milk extrinsic sugars
Non-milk extrinsic sugars	Extrinsic sugars, except lactose, in milk and milk products. Non-milk extrinsic sugars are considered to a be a major contributor to the development of dental caries.
NSP	Non-starch polysaccharides. A precisely measurable compound of food. A measure of 'dietary fibre'.
PUFA	Polyunsaturated fatty acid
RNI	The Reference Nutrient Intake for protein or a vitamin or a mineral. An amount of the nutrient that is enough, or more than enough, for about 97% of the people in a group. If average intake of a group is at the RNI, then the risk of deficiency in the group is small.
WHO	World Health Organisation

Related publications & websites

SOURCE PUBLICATIONS

Department of Health (1991). *Dietary Reference Values: A Guide.*
London, HMSO (now The Stationery Office)

Department of Health (1994). *Report of the Cardiovascular Review Group Committee on Medical Aspects of Food Policy. Nutritional Aspects of Cardiovascular Disease. Report on Health and Social Subjects, No. 46.*
London, HMSO (now The Stationery Office)

Department of Health (1998). *Report of the Subgroup on Bone Health, Working Group on the Nutritional Status of the Population of the Committee on Medical Aspects of Food and Nutrition Policy. Nutrition and Bone Health. Report on Health and Social Subjects, No. 49.*
London, The Stationery Office

Department of Health (1998). *Report of the Working Group on Diet and Cancer of the Committee on Medical Aspects of Food and Nutrition Policy. Nutritional Aspects of the Development of Cancer. Report on Health and Social Subjects, No. 48.*
London, The Stationery Office

Department of Health (1999). *Saving Lives: Our Healthier Nation.* London, The Stationery Office

Department of Health (2000). *The NHS Plan.*
London, The Stationery Office

Ministry of Agriculture, Fisheries and Food (1995). *Manual of Nutrition. 10th Edition.*
London, The Stationery Office

The Royal Society of Chemistry and Ministry of Agriculture, Fisheries and Food (1991). McCance and Widdowson's *The Composition of Foods.* Fifth Edition.
London, The Stationery Office

USEFUL PUBLICATIONS

Eating Well for Older People with Dementia
Published by VOICES
ISBN 0 9532626 0X
Looks at how dementia affects the ability to eat well. Examines the role that good nutrition can play in the care of older people. Provides practical and nutritional guidelines for residential and nursing homes and others catering for older people with dementia. Available from: The Caroline Walker Trust (1998).

Heartbeat Award: a Caterer's Guide to Achieving the Heartbeat Award
ISBN 0 7521 0734 8
A guide for caterers on the background to the heartbeat award explaining how establishments may apply and offering guidance on achieving the award. Available from: Marston Book Services (2000).

The Education (Nutritional Standards for Schools Lunches) (England) Regulations (2000) SI 2000 No. 1777.
ISBN 0 11 099519 X
Details of the compulsory nutritional standards for school lunches to be introduced from April 2001 (see also guidance for caterers on implementation).
Available from: The Stationery Office.

School Nutrition Action Group (SNAG) Newsletter & Training & Resources
ISBN 0 11 099519 X
This information can be obtained from Joe Harvey, The Health Education Trust, 18 High Street, Broom, Alcester, Warks B50 4HJ.
(Please send a large sae with a £1.00 stamp on it)

Catering for Health
Published FSA and DOH
PO Box 369, Hayes, Middlesex UB3 1UT

USEFUL ADDRESSES

(The) Anaphylaxis Campaign
2 Clockhouse Road,
Farnborough, Hampshire GU14 7QY
Tel: 01252 542029
www.anaphylaxis.org.uk

The British Heart Foundation
www.bhf.org.uk

British Meat Nutrition Education Service
www.meatandhealth.com

British Nutrition Foundation
High Holborn House,
52-54 High Holborn,
London WC1V 6RQ
Tel: 020 7404 6504
Fax: 020 7404 6747
Email: postbox@nutrition.org.uk
www.nutrition.org.uk

Coeliac UK
www.coeliac.co.uk

The Dairy Council
164 Shaftesbury Avenue, London WC2H 8HL
Tel: 020 7395 4030
www.milk.co.uk

Department for Education and Skills
Mowden Hall, Staindrop Road,
Darlington DL3 9BG
www.dfes.gov.uk

Department of Health
PO Box 410
Wetherby, Yorkshire LS23 7LN
Tel: 020 7210 4850
www.doh.gov.uk

Diabetes UK
10 Queen Anne Street,
London W1M 0BD
Tel: 020 7323 1531
Fax: 020 7637 3544
www.diabetes.org.uk

Food Standards Agency
Aviation House, 125 Kingsway,
London WC2B 6NH
Tel: 020 7276 8000
www.foodstandards.gov.uk

Health Development Agency
(replaced the Health Education Authority)
Holborn Gate, 330 High Holborn
London WC1V 7BA
Tel: 020 7430 0850
Fax: 020 7061 3390
www.hda.nhs.uk

NHS Estates
(an agency of the Department of Health.
Contact for guidelines on hospital catering)
1 Trevelyan Square,
Boar Lane, Leeds LS1 6AF
Tel: 0113 254 7182
www.nhsestates.gov.uk

The Osteoporosis Society
www.nos.org.uk

The Royal Society for the Promotion of Health
RSH House, 38A St.George's Drive,
London SW1V 4BH
Tel: 020 7630 0121
www.rsph.org

The Royal Institute of Public Health
28 Portland Place,
London W1B 1DE
Tel: 020 7291 8350
www.riph.org.uk

Sustain Food Poverty Network
94 White Lion Street,
London N1 9PF
Tel: 020 7837 1228
www.sustainweb.org

FURTHER INFORMATION
The Balance of Good Health
A pictorial representation of the recommended
balance of diet can also be obtained from the
FSA.

Index